The Managerial School

D0027478

The relationship between welfare and the state has undergone a sustained process of reconfiguration over the past two decades and managerialism has played a key role in this process. In education, parents are now seen as consumers and schools as small businesses, their income dependent on their success in attracting customers within competitive local markets. At the same time, management practices borrowed from business – such as target setting and performance monitoring – now play a key role in regulating schools.

What kinds of schools are the reforms producing? What impact are they having on school culture and values? What are the social justice implications of applying a business model to the provision of schooling?

In *The Managerial School*, Sharon Gewirtz draws on in-depth interviews with teachers in a range of secondary schools and close observation of school practices to answer these questions. Through a comparison of Conservative and New Labour policies, she argues that New Labour's 'third way' for education is a contradictory mix of neo-liberal, authoritarian and humanistic strands that is not in any real sense a new educational settlement.

This empirically based account of over a decade of education reform offers a unique insight into the effects of managerialism on schools and a hard-hitting analysis of the inherent tensions in a system that undoubtedly perpetrates social injustice.

Sharon Gewirtz is Professor of Education at King's College London.

The State of Welfare
Edited by Mary Langan

Throughout the Western world, welfare states are in transition. Changing social, economic and political circumstances have rendered obsolete the systems that emerged in the 1940s out of the experiences of depression, war and social conflict. New structures of welfare are now taking shape in response to the conditions of today: globalisation and individuation, the demise of traditional allegiances and institutions, the rise of new forms of identity and solidarity.

In Britain, the New Labour government has linked the projects of implementing a new welfare settlement and forging a new moral purpose in society. Enforcing 'welfare to work', on the one hand, and tackling 'social exclusion', on the other, the government aims to rebalance the rights and duties of citizens and redefine the concept of equality.

The State of Welfare series provides a forum for the debate about the new shape of welfare into the millennium.

Titles of related interest also in *The State of Welfare* series:

The Managerial School

Post-welfarism and Social Justice
in Education

Sharon Gewirtz

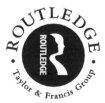

London and New York

First published 2002
by Routledge
11 New Fetter Lane, London EC4P 4EE

Simultaneously published in the USA and Canada
by Routledge
29 West 35th Street, New York, NY 10001

Routledge is an imprint of the Taylor & Francis Group

© 2002 Sharon Gewirtz

Typeset in Times by BC Typesetting, Bristol
Printed and bound in Great Britain by
TJ International Ltd, Padstow, Cornwall

All rights reserved. No part of this book may be reprinted or reproduced
or utilised in any form or by any electronic, mechanical, or other means,
now known or hereafter invented, including photocopying and
recording, or in any information storage or retrieval system, without
permission in writing from the publishers.

British Library Cataloguing in Publication Data
A catalogue record for this book is available from the British Library

Library of Congress Cataloging in Publication Data
Gewirtz, Sharon, 1964–
    The managerial school: post-welfarism and social justice in education/
    Sharon Gewirtz.
        p.   cm. – (The state of welfare)
    Includes bibliographical references and index.
    1. School management and organization–Great Britain.
    2. Educational change–Great Britain. 3. Great Britain–Social
    policy. I. Title. II. Series.
    LB2900.5.G49 2001
    371.2'00941–dc21   2001019454

ISBN 0–415–22485–3 (hbk)
ISBN 0–415–22486–1 (pbk)

For Gáti

Contents

List of tables

Preface

The 1988 Education Reform Act fundamentally transformed the organisation of school provision in England and Wales. This major piece of legislation redefined parents as consumers, who – at least in principle – were given the right to choose a school for their child, rather than be allocated one by local authority bureaucrats. At the same time, schools were effectively reconfigured as small businesses whose income was to become dependent on their success in attracting customers within competitive local school markets. These were not free markets, however, as various mechanisms were put in place by the 1988 Act to enable a tight regulation of schooling by the state. In particular, the 1988 Act gave central government the right to specify precisely what was to be taught in schools and to monitor closely the performance of schools through the national curriculum, regular testing of students, the publication of those results and inspection. Since the 1988 legislation, a series of further reforms have consolidated and extended the marketisation and regulation of school provision. The New Labour government, first elected in 1997, appears to have adopted a more humanistic approach to the curriculum than their Conservative predecessors, who had been responsible for the 1988 Act. It has also sought to introduce a degree of compensatory funding for (some) socially distressed areas and uses the language of partnership and collaboration rather than competition. Nevertheless, in a number of crucial respects, New Labour policies represent a continuation of the Conservatives' crusade to make the provision of education more business-like.

The essays collected together here are about the effects that this business model of education provision is having on schools in England and, more particularly, on the culture and values which pervade them. What kinds of schools are the reforms producing? Who and what is valued in them? What impact are the reforms having on the roles of headteachers and teachers, on how they think and talk about their work and on the nature of relationships inside schools? What are the social justice implications of applying business-like modes of organisation and management to the provision of schooling? And how compatible are these new modes of provision with the seemingly humanistic and social democratic educational commitments espoused by New Labour?

Throughout the book, the term 'welfarism' is used to represent the educational 'settlement' – i.e., the sets of languages, meanings, assumptions, values and institutional forms, practices and relationships – which framed the organisation of schooling between 1944 and 1988. And the term 'post-welfarism' is used to refer to the settlement inaugurated by the New Right-inspired reforms of the 1980s and 1990s. The shift from welfarism to post-welfarism is less clear cut and is messier in practice than the neatness that the labelling might suggest and some of this messiness will become apparent as the book develops. Nevertheless, I want to argue that there are important features that distinguish the post-1988 period from the preceding era. For the sake of convenience, the terms 'welfarism' and 'post-welfarism' are used to capture these two distinct phases and to signify the range of shifts in language, practices, purposes and values which have accompanied the drive to make schools more business-like.

Chapter 1 sets the scene for the book. It begins by sketching out the main policy components of the shift from welfarism to post-welfarism and the conditions out of which this shift arose, drawing attention to key problems of the state that post-welfarist policies were meant to help remedy – problems of capital accumulation, social control and legitimation. Chapter 1 then goes on to outline the rationale and approach of the book, which is rooted in a critique of two dominant trends in research on education policy and practice. The first trend, which I refer to as the celebration-of-indeterminacy approach, is influenced by particular variants of post-modernist thought. The second is the growing and increasingly influential body of research into what has become known as 'school effectiveness and improvement'. Whilst rooted within two very different epistemological traditions, both trends, I argue – albeit for different reasons – effectively underplay the extent to which state policies and the discursive and socio-economic contexts within which schools operate, constrain and shape what goes on in schools. The chapter concludes by arguing for an approach to the analysis of post-welfarism in education that overcomes the pitfalls of these trends. I suggest that we need to make use of insights from neo-Marxism, whilst not losing sight of the contribution that post-modernist theory can make to our understanding of policies and their effects.

Part I of the book, post-welfarism and the reconstruction of English schooling, examines the implications of post-welfarism for the culture, values and relations of secondary schooling. Culture is conceptualised in a very broad and simple sense to refer to the ways in which people think, act and communicate, to 'the material and symbolic artifacts of behaviour' (Thomas 1993: 12) (for example, methods of grouping students, school prospectuses, school uniforms) and to the meanings signified by behaviour and its artefacts. In this part of the book, ethnographic data are used to explore what managerialism means for headteachers, teachers and students working in a range of socio-economic contexts.[1]

The research upon which the chapters in Part I draw was conducted in London schools. However, whilst it is important to recognise that London schools may have distinctive features, the insights developed from this research have, I would suggest, a wider applicability. The schools which took part in the research were chosen deliberately as critical cases to enable an exploration of what is happening in schools that are located in *an archetypically post-welfarist environment* – i.e., one where quasi-markets operate. And the cultural and value effects reported here are ones that will no doubt be familiar to those involved in schools in other parts of England, as well as in other countries where similar policies have been adopted. Certainly, there is now a growing body of research emanating from various parts of the world which appears to confirm some of the key findings reported here. (See Whitty *et al.* 1998 for a useful overview of research into school reform in England and Wales, the USA, Australia, New Zealand and Sweden.)

One of the consequences of post-welfarist policies in education has been to draw attention to, and enhance the role of, the headteacher and, since headteachers play a key part in shaping their school's response to the new policy environment, in any analysis of cultural and value change in schools a focus on the headteacher is vital. Chapter 2, therefore, considers shifts in the languages and practices of school headship. The chapter is grounded in an analysis of one school which, I suggest, is a critical case because it brings into sharp focus the discursive shift that a number of commentators have noted is evident on a larger scale in the education and welfare system as a whole. However, by focusing on the contingent and the local, the chapter also illustrates the varied and complex ways in which individual

---

1 See Appendix for details of the research methods used in the two studies upon which Part I is based.

headteachers may position themselves within the shifting organisational and discursive terrains in which they are located.

Chapter 3 explores the ways in which the education market functions as a system of rewards and punishments, a disciplinary mechanism, fostering particular cultural forms and socio-psychological dispositions and marginalising others. The chapter considers the case of a school that has had to confront the issue of institutional survival in a market context. The resulting value conflicts and ethical dilemmas faced by the staff and governors are discussed.

Chapter 4 explores the effects upon teachers of post-welfarist education policies, as mediated by the new discourses and policies of school managers. More specifically, it is concerned with the emotional, relational and pedagogical aspects of teachers' work. The chapter describes how the pressures created by managerialist discourses and the market environment – in particular, heightened forms of competition, assessment, surveillance and performance monitoring, and the intensification of the labour process of teaching – have led to demoralisation amongst teachers and to perceptions of a decline in collaboration and the erosion of creativity in classroom practice.

Chapter 5 challenges a central strand of managerialist thinking in education that so-called failing schools are largely the product of poor leadership and teaching and that, through the 'cascading of best practice', all schools can be a success. Drawing on ethnographic data from two schools, the chapter demonstrates the intricate and intimate connections between what school managers and teachers do and the socio-economic and discursive environments within which they operate.

Whilst Part I of the book uses case studies to explore specific aspects of post-welfarist schooling, Part II, Assessing post-welfarism in Education, 'stands back' from these studies. Part II attempts to draw together the threads of the analysis in Part I in order to make a broader assessment of the characteristics and consequences of educational post-welfarism and to speculate about the likely consequences of New Labour's 'third way' for education.

Chapter 6 begins by emphasising the complexity of the 'lived' post-welfarist settlement, and its contested nature and warning against the twin dangers of over-generalisation and 'golden-ageism'. It then goes on to identify the key features of post-welfarism in education. It is suggested that these define the contours within and against which diverse responses are articulated. The chapter concludes by arguing that post-welfarism is failing to ameliorate the problems it was meant to help solve and that it contains its own tensions and contradictions.

Using a conceptualisation of social justice, which has at its heart a recognition of the importance of diverse cultural identities, Chapter 7 presents a social justice 'audit' of post-welfarism in education. In this chapter, it is argued that the post-welfarist policies introduced by successive Conservative governments seems to have contributed to a regressive redistribution of educational resources and to have generated a number of forms of oppression – notably, an intensified exploitation of teachers, the increased marginalisation of working-class students and some racialised groups, and the circumscription of opportunities for the development of pedagogies that recognise and engage with diverse cultural identities.

Chapter 8 considers New Labour's 'third way' for education, which, it is argued, comprises a contradictory mix of neo-liberal, authoritarian and humanistic strands. This final chapter draws upon the analysis of earlier chapters to speculate about the consequences of 'third way' policies for social justice, whether they represent a new educational settlement or a consolidation of post-welfarism and how far these policies are likely to resolve the tensions associated with the Conservative reforms.

The emphasis throughout this book is upon critique. This is because, whilst in particular settings managerialism may represent a field of constraints *and* possibilities (Clarke and Newman 1997: 104–5), the evidence upon which this book is based strongly suggests that within school settings the constraining features of managerialism tend to predominate – although as we shall see, these constraining features do not operate uniformly across different material and socio-economic contexts.

Acknowledgements

This book draws upon research into post-welfarism in education carried out over a ten-year period and it owes much to collaborative work with, and the support of, colleagues at King's College London and the Open University with whom I have worked during this time.

The project started in 1990 when I began work as a researcher at King's College London on a study funded by the UK Economic and Social Research Council (ESRC) (award no. R000232858) that looked at the operation and effects of markets in education in the wake of the 1988 Education Reform Act. I am indebted to the directors of that project, Stephen Ball and Richard Bowe, for giving me a job which enabled me to develop my interest in markets in education and for inducting me into fruitful and stimulating ways of doing collaborative research. Many of the arguments developed in this book were inspired initially by this joint work and Chapter 3 is adapted from an article that was originally published in all our names. I am grateful to Stephen and Richard for allowing me to use this article here. The markets research led to a second ESRC-funded study (award no. R000235544), which I co-directed with Stephen Ball. This study focused on the impact of market forces on the culture and values of schooling. Chapters 2, 4 and 5 draw on fieldwork and were inspired by conversations carried out as part of that study. Chapter 2 is an amended version of an article first published in our joint names, and I am grateful to Stephen for giving me permission to include it in this book. Thanks are also due to Diane Reay, who carried out some of the interviews in two of the case-study schools, to the ESRC for funding both studies, and to all the school governors and staff who participated in the studies. I am particularly grateful to the chair of governors at 'Northwark Park' school who read and commented on Chapter 3 and to the headteacher of 'Fletcher' school and the head of religious education at 'Beatrice Webb' school who commented on an earlier version of Chapter 4.

This book also draws on thinking and writing I did as part of my PhD and I would like to thank Stephen Ball (again) and Geoff Whitty for the excellent advice and support they gave me in their capacity as joint supervisors of my thesis. My external examiner, Michael Apple, also made extremely helpful comments that I have tried to take on board.

There are other colleagues whose support has been invaluable. Alan Cribb, Meg Maguire and Chiz Dubé at King's have been good friends to me over the last decade. Alan has read endless drafts, helped me to clarify my thinking, has been a great source of moral support, and has generally exhibited saint-like qualities. Meg has also read drafts and remains a constant source of inspiration and encouragement. And I am grateful to Chiz for transcribing many of the interviews drawn upon in this book. Liz Cawdron and Helen Worger have provided excellent transcriptions as well and I am most appreciative of their work.

This book also owes much to the support of colleagues in the Social Policy Discipline at the Open University, who have for the last three years provided me with an incredibly warm, lively and inspiring context within which to work. I would particularly like to thank John Clarke who has given generously of his time and wisdom, reading and commenting on drafts of several chapters, Gail Lewis who read and helped improve an earlier draft of Chapter 7 and has helped stimulate my thinking more generally, Gordon Hughes who has managed to find time in his hectic schedule to read and provide useful feedback on other parts of this book, and Sue Lacey, Pauline Hetherington, Donna Collins and Nicole Jones for their brilliant secretarial support.

Early drafts of some of the chapters of this book were aired at meetings of the 'Parental Choice and Market Forces' group held at King's College London and I am grateful to all the participants in these discussions, some of whom have already been mentioned. The others are Gill Crozier, Miriam David, John Fitz, David Halpin, Hugh Lauder, Philip Noden, Sally Power, Carol Vincent and Anne West. I am particularly grateful to Carol for her very helpful comments on Chapters 6, 7 and 8.

Last, but definitely not least, this book could not have been written without the ongoing support of my partner, Desmond O'Reilly, my three children, Flynn, Freda and Eva, and my friends, Jude Lancet and Carrie Supple.

Most of the chapters in this volume are revised versions of articles published elsewhere or contain portions of articles published elsewhere.

Sections of Chapter 1 and Chapter 6 originally appeared in 'Efficiency at any cost', in C. Symes and D. Meadmore (eds) (1999), *The Extraordinary School*, Peter Lang.

Chapter 2 is a revised version of 'From "Welfarism" to "New Manageririalism" : shifting discourses of school headship in the education marketplace', *Discourse* 21(3) (2000) (co-authored with Stephen Ball).

Chapter 3 is a revised version of 'Values and ethics in the Education Marketplace: the case of Northwark Park', *International Studies in Sociology of Education* 3(2) (1994) (co-authored with Stephen Ball and Richard Bowe).

Chapter 4 is revised from an article originally published in the *Journal of Education Policy* 12(4) (1997), entitled 'Post-welfarism and the reconstruction of teachers' work in the UK'.

Chapter 5 is a revised version of an article published in the *Oxford Review of Education* 2(4) (1998).

Chapter 7 is revised from an article published in *Education and Social Justice* 1 (1998) and a chapter in G. Lewis, S. Gewirtz and J. Clarke (eds) (2000) *Rethinking Social Policy*, Sage.

Finally, Chapter 8 draws on material from 'Education Action Zones: emblems of the "third way"?', in H. Dean and R. Woods (eds) (1999) *Social Policy Review 11*, SPA and 'Bringing the Politics back in: a critical analysis of quality discourses in education', *British Journal of Educational Studies* 48(4) (2000).

1 Introduction

The changing politics of education: from welfarism to post-welfarism

This introductory chapter sets out the policy context and rationale for the book as a whole. It begins by describing the key components of the shift from welfarism to post-welfarism, the assumptions underpinning the post-welfarist settlement and the conditions out of which the shift arose. The chapter then goes on to outline the book's analytical approach.

From the mid-1940s to the mid-1980s, the English schools system was broadly shaped by an ideology and set of languages, policies and practices which together made up what can loosely be categorised as a *welfarist* settlement. The term settlement is used here to refer to the specific constellation of assumptions and arrangements – political, economic, social and institutional – which framed school provision during this period. The welfarist settlement was underpinned by a broad consensus amongst powerful groups – the major political parties, the trade unions and big business – and by a significant degree of popular support. However, contestation, conflict and fragility are defining features of all settlements – they can only ever represent a temporary 'equilibrium' (Gramsci 1971) – and the welfarist settlement in education was no exception. The instabilities of the welfarist settlement, which gave rise to the emergence of post-welfarist policies, practices and values, will be examined later in the chapter but first I want to identify the key policy components of the shift from welfarism to post-welfarism.

Welfarism entailed a formal commitment to distributive justice; that is, to the redistribution of social goods on a more equitable basis. It was grounded in the economics of Keynesianism and the politics of corporatism and was underpinned by the 'social democratic consensus' (CCCS 1981). I say *formal* commitment because, of course, in practice, welfarism failed to eradicate enormous social inequalities – although it might have had an ameliorative effect for some – and the label corporatism thinly veils the unequal power relations between the 'partners'. The major policy manifestations of welfarism within the field of secondary schooling were the expansion of 'secondary education for all' and bipartism in the immediate post-war period (sometimes referred to as the meritocratic phase), followed by the introduction of comprehensive schooling and the raising of the school leaving age (the comprehensive phase). Corporatism in education was characterised by a 'partnership' between the central state, the local education authorities and the teacher unions.

In the welfarist era, welfare work was governed by what John Clarke and Janet Newman have called two 'modes of coordination' – bureaucratic administration and professionalism – or 'bureau-professionalism'. By mode of coordination they mean:

> the complex of rules, roles and regulatory principles around which the social practices of organisations are structured – which generate typical patterns of internal and external social relationships and which, among other things, privilege certain types of knowledge.
>
> (Clarke and Newman 1997: 5)

Within the schools system, bureaucratic administration and professionalism both had key roles to play in coordinating provision. The institutional locus of bureaucratic administration was the local education authority (LEA). Here, rules and procedures to govern such things as the allocation of resources, the building and maintenance of schools, and the organisation of school meals, transport and admissions were generated within a hierarchical framework. But professionalism also had an important part to play in the LEAs where teams of experts – for example, educational psychologists, welfare officers, advisors and inspectors – were based. Moreover, education officers were not 'just' administrators. Having been a teacher was a prerequisite for employment as an education officer and officers played a significant role in providing support and expertise to teachers, for example, through staff development services. In schools, teachers operated as relatively autonomous professionals, with the head as leading professional and 'senior architect' of the school's curriculum (Fergusson 1994: 102).

In the *post-welfarist* era the formal commitments to Keynesian economics and distributive justice were dropped and replaced by formal commitments to market 'democracy' and competitive individualism. Key welfarist orthodoxies were challenged, in particular the view that

welfare was best provided within bureaucratic organisational formations. Now welfare bureaucrats and professionals were held to be the
source of major problems rather than the source of solutions. They
were branded as inefficient, self-interested and guilty of fostering
welfare dependency and undermining the self-reliance of their clients.

The legislative manifestation of post-welfarism in education is a set
of policies which, as shorthand, are referred to throughout this book
as the *post-welfarist education policy complex* (PWEPC). The PWEPC
is comprised of a number of disparate elements that initially emerged
out of different ideological traditions and pragmatic concerns within
the Conservative Party. However, as we shall see, the New Labour
government first elected in 1997 not only retained but also added to
the complex. I call these disparate (and at times apparently contradictory) elements a complex because of the way they combine to produce specific effects, in particular, the exertion of a greater degree of
state control over schools, colleges, universities, teachers and lecturers,
within a context of devolved management. The key elements of the
complex that relate to the schools sector in the Conservative era
(1979–97) are set out in Table 1.

In addition to discourses of choice and diversity, the complex is
permeated by a utilitarian discourse of efficiency, effectiveness, performance and productivity. Its elements combine to constrain schools and
teachers whilst increasing central control over the school system. First,
the abolition of secondary picketing and teachers' negotiating rights
constitute mechanisms for depressing wages. Second, the PWEPC
has given agents within the state an enhanced capacity to define the
content and desired outcomes of education through the national curriculum, testing and the standardisation of initial teacher training.
And third, through Ofsted (Office for Standards in Education), the
market and performance tables, the PWEPC has enabled the state
to *attempt* to ensure that those outcomes are attained in the most
efficient ways. In this context, the market mechanism is meant to function as a system of resource allocation in which resources flow away
from 'low-performance' (unpopular) schools and towards 'high-
performance' (popular) ones. The system was designed in part to ensure
that only minimal funds are spent on schools that are under-
performing, and where schools are seriously under-performing (i.e.,
'failing') Ofsted can set in motion moves to close or amalgamate
them. Within schools, the efficient use of resources is encouraged by
devolving to headteachers control over their own budgets and by giving
them a financial incentive, through *per capita* funding, to spend resources
in ways which will lead to improved performance.

Table 1 Key school-related elements of the post-welfarist education policy complex, 1979–97

Key school-related elements	Legislation
Abolition of secondary industrial action	1980 Employment Act
Removal of teachers' negotiating rights, imposition of new teaching contracts and new pay and promotional structures	1987 and 1991 Teachers' Pay and Conditions Acts
National curriculum, national testing at four 'key stages' and performance tables	1988 Education Reform Act
Local management of schools and *per capita* funding	1988 Education Reform Act
Parental 'choice' (open enrolment) and 'diversity' (i.e., new types of school, e.g., grant-maintained schools, city technology colleges and other specialist schools). Increased representation of parents on governing bodies. *The Parent's Charter* (DES 1991; DFE 1994a)	1980, 1986, 1988 and 1993 Education Acts
Ofsted and the new inspection regime	1992 Education (Schools) Act
Establishment of Council for the Accreditation of Teacher Education and subsequently Teacher Training Agency to oversee teacher training, and publication of centrally determined criteria upon which approval of courses is based	Circulars 3/84, 9/92 and 14/93 and 1994 Education Act
Each governing body required to set performance targets for its pupils in all public examinations and key-stage assessments and make them public	1997 Education Act

These reforms were accompanied by a 'discourse of derision' (Ball 1990a) that was mobilised against teachers and local authority bureaucrats, in an effort to manufacture a new common sense in support of post-welfarist policies. As Ross Fergusson explains:

> Teachers were denigrated as self-interested and unaccountable. And while self-interest is normalized as part of the discourse of market relations, and elsewhere is celebrated as the engine of progress, it is seen in this instance as invalidating teachers' claims to professionalism. Other routes to breaking bureau professional power entailed the public questioning of the competency of teachers, allegations of the failure of the comprehensive system, the down-skilling of teachers' professional knowledge through the exclusion of theory in favour of more instrumental forms of initial training and in-service staff development . . . Local education authorities came under attack as part of the wider attack on local democracy. . . . They were said to be part of the bureau-professional power bloc, controlling the character of local schools, causing high public spending, and imposing 'politicized' values which challenged some of the key assumptions of social relations and normalities.
>
> (Fergusson 1998: 230)

Bureaucratic modes of coordination were held to be both ineffective and inflexible, as the US academics, Chubb and Moe, passionate advocates of choice in education, explain:

> Bureaucracy vitiates the most basic requirements of effective organization. It imposes goals, structures, and requirements that tell principals and teachers what to do and how to do it – denying them not only the discretion they need to exercise their expertise and professional judgement but also the flexibility they need to develop and operate as teams. The key to effective education rests with unleashing the productive potential already present in the schools and their personnel. It rests with granting them the autonomy to do what they do best . . . [T]he freer schools are from external control the more likely they are to have effective organizations.
>
> (Chubb and Moe 1990: 187)

Somewhat paradoxically, given the constraints imposed by the national curriculum, testing and a stringent inspection regime, the

PWEPC was designed, at least in part, to 'unleash the productive potential' of school managers whilst constraining what were seen as the stultifying bureaucratic procedures and attitudes of LEAs. The idea was that by giving headteachers and governors control over their budgets and by making school income dependent on attracting custom, senior managers in schools would have both the tools and the incentive to behave in more cost-effective, flexible, competitive, consumer-satisfying and innovative ways. One of the key rationales underpinning the reforms, then, was that market forces and more efficient management techniques would help raise standards in schools. The underlying assumption was that if schools were given autonomy to respond to market forces (within the broad constraints set by the national curriculum, national testing and Ofsted's inspection criteria) then any failure to improve and boost recruitment could be blamed on poor management and teaching.

It was in accordance with such thinking that corporate and bureau-professional modes of coordination were undermined and in their place attempts made to erect new managerial regimes. The essential differences between the archetypal professional/bureaucrat and the archetypal new manager are succinctly captured by Clarke and Newman as follows:

> By contrast with the professional, the manager is customer focused and is driven by the search for efficiency rather than abstract 'professional standards'. Compared to the bureaucrat, the manager is flexible and outward looking. Unlike the politician, the manager inhabits the 'real world' of 'good business practices' not the realms of doctrinaire ideology . . . The significance of management as a regime lies in the claim that managers 'do the right things'. It is this which underpins management as a mode of power and is associated with an insistent demand that managers must be given the 'freedom' or the 'right to manage'.
>
> (Clarke and Newman 1992a: 6)

The PWEPC demands the realignment of school practices to performance criteria set by the state and managerialism is the device which has evolved to effect this realignment, in particular through the strategies of target-setting, performance monitoring and a closer surveillance of teachers. Crucially, the PWEPC exists within a wider economic and policy environment which itself constrains teachers and makes a powerful contribution to the restructuring of their work. First, in periods of high unemployment, 'the dull compulsion of economic relations' (Marx 1976) is likely to constitute, for many teachers, an enormous incentive to acquiesce to the pressures of post-welfarism. In addition, the increase in poverty generated by labour market restructuring, unemployment and the wider post-welfarist policy complex (Hills 1995; Piachaud 1999) places enormous pressures and constraints on the work of schools and teachers within them.

However, the shift from welfarism to post-welfarism has, of course, not been as neat and tidy as my account so far might suggest and the boundaries between the two eras are blurred. For example, as Clarke and colleagues (1994: 5) have pointed out, 'managerialism in the public sector has a confused and contradictory political history'. Indeed Clarke *et al.* suggest that some of the public sector management theories which came to dominate in the late 1980s and 1990s may have had their roots in the practices and thinking of the new urban left councils of the early 1980s. Furthermore, market forces and managerial modes of coordination were not simply and unproblematically imposed on a passive and undifferentiated work force. The processes and practices of markets and managerialism have been variously welcomed, agonised over, contested and reworked by public sector managers and workers, and the impact of managerialism has been – and indeed continues to be – uneven (Clarke *et al.* 1994, 2000). Nevertheless, as we shall see, it is no doubt the case that post-welfarist policies have altered significantly the conditions within which public-sector workers in general and teachers in particular operate, forcing them to respond in some way, whether by enthusiastic compliance, reluctant implication, subversion or outright resistance.

But how do we begin to explain the emergence of the PWEPC? First of all, it is important to recognise that the English educational policies of the 1980s and 1990s were not unique. Similar policies have been advocated and introduced in other countries – for example, Sweden, the USA, Canada, Australia and New Zealand – across a whole range of public-sector services (Whitty *et al.* 1998). The ideological roots of managerialism in education can be seen in part to lie in critiques of business management by US economists in the late 1970s and 1980s. The central plank of these criticisms was that business managers, operating within inflexible and over-regulated corporations and within an over-interventionist state, were inefficient, uninnovative and uncompetitive. The answer lay in a free-market economy, the reassertion of the 'managerial prerogative' or 'the manager's right to manage', the marginalisation of trade unions and new management techniques (like Total Quality Management and Human Resource

Management). Those arguments were in turn adopted within some sections of British industry as well as by New Right politicians:

> At the level of political debate, the New Right presented a new view of British management as well as its traditional pejorative focus on the trade unions. Though the latter were clearly identified with considerable inefficiencies in the operation of the labour market, British managers were also seen as contributing to the poor performance of the British economy. Initiatives were devised which would enhance the professionalism of British managers and improve their training and educational credentials . . . To achieve a level of international parity management needed to be understood as a strategic activity demonstrating a proactive capacity, a reversal of the 1970s image where a corporatist environment had denuded much of its entrepreneurial space. Behind many of these developments lay a commitment to re-establish an unfettered market economy where management could take the initiative; planning, controlling and co-ordinating the factors of production. Less constrained decisions could be made which more closely reflected codes of business efficiency and were particularly related to the specific needs of individual companies . . .
>
> (Ozga 1995: 9–10)

Subsequently, these same ideas were applied to management in the public sector. Alongside education, health, housing, social work and the criminal justice and benefits systems have all been restructured with a view to altering the culture of welfare provision.

The advocacy of markets in education has a longer history than managerialism and can be traced back to the publication of *The Wealth of Nations* in 1776. In this book, Adam Smith had argued that parents ought to pay at least some of the cost of their children's education directly to the school. If the state were to foot the entire bill, he suggested, the teacher 'would soon learn to neglect his business' (Smith 1937). Subsequently, a kind of proto-voucher was advocated by Tom Paine in *The Rights of Man*. However, contemporary proposals for 'social markets' are rooted in Hayekian neo-liberalism. Friedrich Hayek's (1944) arguments for the decentralisation of economic and social decision-making were taken up and developed in relation to education by one of his Chicago acolytes, the economist Milton Friedman in an article, 'The role of government in education', published in 1955. The article was reproduced and more widely disseminated in Friedman's classic *Capitalism and Freedom* (1962), and his proposals subsequently taken on board in England, where a series of pamphlets by New Right libertarians were published. Like Friedman, these English pamphleteers advocated the market as the best 'device for registering individual preferences and allocating resources to satisfy them' (Harris and Seldon 1979: 5; see also Harris 1969; Boyson 1975; Cox and Boyson 1977; Sexton 1987). The principle of consumer sovereignty, they urged, should be paramount. That principle holds:

> that each individual is the best judge of his or her needs and wants and of what is in their best interests. If there is some mechanism through which consumers can accurately express their preferences, and if there is a system of incentives for producers to respond to them, then resources will be directed away from activities which do not satisfy consumers to those which do.
>
> (Ashworth, Papps and Thomas 1988: 4)

Markets in education are supported by neo-liberals not only on economic grounds (i.e., that choice will ensure that consumers – usually parents, sometimes industry, but rarely children – get what they want and will raise standards in the most efficient way possible). But they are also advocated on ethical grounds. Greater freedom for parents to choose schools and for managers to manage them is viewed as an intrinsically good thing because, as John Gray has put it, autonomy is 'one of the vital ingredients of individual well-being in the modern world' (1992: 2). There are some libertarians who also argue that choice will lead to a fairer distribution of educational resources. It is suggested that in the system that operated in England before 1988, where school places were allocated largely on the basis of catchment areas (i.e., where students lived), better-off families were privileged. This is because the better off could afford to buy houses in areas where the schools were thought to be superior. This is what Kenneth Clarke, former Conservative Secretary of State for Education, dubbed 'selection by mortgage':

> The way in which Labour made our schools comprehensive from the 1960s onwards damaged opportunities very seriously for children from poor families in deprived parts of our cities. Selection by mortgage replaced selection by examination and the eleven plus route was closed for many bright working-class boys and girls.
>
> (Clarke 1991: 2–3)

Proponents of markets in education claim that the choice mechanism does not discriminate on the basis of socio-economic status – it is 'class-blind'.

Arguments for devolution and choice in education were also taken up by some on the conservative New Right. On the surface, this appears somewhat paradoxical, given the hostility of neo-conservatives towards the liberal notion of individual autonomy. However, for the neo-conservative think tank, the Hillgate Group, the 'restoration' of traditionalism in schools (i.e., respect for the family, private property and authority) could only be achieved if schools were liberated from the control of local authorities, who needed to be deprived of 'their standing ability to corrupt the minds and soul of the young' (Hillgate Group 1986: 18).

Having sketched out some of the ideological lineages of managerialism and markets in education, I now want to consider why it was that from the mid–1970s these philosophies of educational governance came to be accepted within Conservative Party circles and subsequently came to govern policy-making.

The reasons for the breakdown of the welfarist settlement in education and for the attempts to transport management practices and market economics from the private to the public sector are complicated. However, the most convincing explanations situate an analysis of struggles over policy, within and across the state and civil society, in the context of an analysis of the problems which agents within the state feel a need to resolve (CCCS 1981; Dale 1989; Ball 1990a). These problems can be divided into three broad categories – problems of capital accumulation, problems of control and problems of legitimation. In what follows, I will briefly set out the nature of the problems and their consequences for education.

There were two major problems of capital accumulation that had direct implications for the welfarist settlement in education. First, the oil crisis of the mid-1970s prompted a fiscal crisis, creating an imperative (or at least a widely perceived imperative) for the reduction of public expenditure in general and education spending in particular. Second, there was a perception that British industry was experiencing a decline in competitiveness. There were (and are) conflicting diagnoses of, and prescriptions for, this decline (Ashton and Green 1996), the most common explanations being economic globalisation and new (post-fordist) forms of production based on modern, knowledge-based forms of technology. However, what is relevant here is not the veracity of the diagnoses or explanations but that perceptions of a decline in the performance of British industry in relation to its international competitors led attention to be focused on the perceived inadequacy of the state education system in preparing young people with appropriate attitudes and skills for employment.

During the late 1960s and 1970s, the state also faced problems of control – symbolised by the student 'unrest' of 1968 and the trebling of the strike rate between 1968 and 1972. *Unpopular Education*, the Centre for Contemporary Cultural Studies' (CCCS 1981) history of schooling and social democracy since 1944, vividly captures how various forms of social conflict and challenge within and beyond schools contributed to the destabilisation of welfarism in education. The CCCS identify at least three sources of social instability. First, the universities were seen to pose a challenge by 'producing not the bright young managers and technicians of a renovated capitalism, but a new disaffected, in whom the work ethic and self-discipline seemed to have been replaced by hedonism and disdain for rationality' (1981: 174).

The second source of instability came from the workforce who 'in no way behaved as had been hoped: that is, as the owners of skills, as the individual capitalists, that human capital theory had expected . . . Rather, large sections of the British workforce behaved, at this time, as dispossessed wage labourers fighting to maintain or increase their share of the value produced' (CCCS 1981: 174–75).

The third source of instability was located within schools. Here there were a number of forces at work. To begin with, many teachers experienced comprehensive re-organisation as unsettling:

> The *ad hoc* nature of [comprehensivisation] made worse by lack of money for new secondary building schemes under the Conservatives, entailed huge organisational difficulties, including split sites and very large schools. For many the actual processes of teaching became more problematic, particularly in a period of heightened consciousness about youth unrest. These changes sometimes meant that teachers and pupils from vastly different traditions were thrown together. As a result, conflicts over discipline, curriculum and the handling of informal school cultures were engendered among teachers and pupils.
>
> (CCCS 1981: 188)

Additional instabilities were generated by the raising of the school leaving age (ROSLA) from September 1973, which increased the proportion of young people in the schools system who were categorised as 'non-academic'. ROSLA thereby contributed to an escalation of 'indiscipline', truancy and student discontent, some of which was channelled into organised social action seen, for example, in the setting up of the National Union of School Students and the movements for children's rights. Although exaggerated by the media, movements of radical teachers also emerged, 'as those involved in the counter-culture and student movements of the late 1960s entered teaching, and took there a concern with the curriculum, often protesting its distance from their own or their pupils' experience, and a concern with social relations inside the classroom and the school as a whole' (CCCS 1981: 189). These radical teacher movements included a strong feminist strand, with women teachers challenging the under-representation of women in senior positions in schools and the taken-for-granted patriarchal assumptions which structured the curriculum.

The CCCS demonstrates how these various conflicts and challenges contributed to the construction, by neo-conservatives and the media, of a moral panic and to calls for more authoritarian modes of control. For the writers of the *Black Papers* (a series of educational essays emanating from the conservative New Right) and of the tabloid newspapers, egalitarian policies and militant teachers were responsible for turning schools into sites of 'defiance, gang war and mugging' (*Sunday People*, June 1974, cited in CCCS 1981: 198). Disorder in schools was also associated in such writings with a decline in academic standards.

At the same time, the state faced escalating problems of legitimation. Welfarism was seen not only to have failed to meet the requirements of capital accumulation and to have contributed to a crisis of control, thus alienating significant sectors of capital and other powerful social groups. It had also failed in one of its central objectives – to produce greater distributive justice – creating a large pool of disaffected working-class and young black people, and hence a crisis of legitimation. As the CCCS put it:

> The brief experience of working-class pupils and parents of reforms which had promised greater progress and equality was not now able to generate support in a period of heightened conflict when schools remained a distant and divisive escalator, out of the class, for the few. The reality of the reproduction of class differentiation was unchanged. New qualifications which had promised upskilling and better employment were proving a debased currency. If anything, the production of new aspirations was as likely to achieve greater resentment at their disappointment.
>
> (CCCS 1981: 176)

The amount of weight that should be given to each set of problems in prompting the destabilisation and decline of the welfarist settlement in education is a contestable issue. But the main point here is that, to some extent, all three problems – of capital accumulation, social control and legitimation – may be seen to have generated a desire amongst policy makers to reduce the power of trade unions and of bureaucrats in the local authorities, and to control more directly the work of managers and teachers in schools. These providers of education were seen to be, not only profligate, but a threat to the competitiveness of British industry and to social order, and responsible, at least in part, for a decline of confidence in the state education system. A major impetus behind the PWEPC, then, was the view that, if faith in the education system and more traditional forms of authority were to be restored, if public expenditure on education was to be reduced and if schools were going to respond effectively to the changing requirements of the economy, then schooling needed to be liberated from the control of teachers and their unions.

Of crucial relevance to this book is the point that in liberating schools from the damaging effects of control by the so-called educational establishment, its workers and their unions, the PWEPC was meant to effect a *re-acculturation* of schooling. The PWEPC had embedded within it a set of beliefs, which in certain respects appear contradictory, about what education was for and about how those who managed and worked in schools should behave. Different fractions within the Conservative Party deemed different forms of cultural change to be necessary. For example, for the 'industrial trainers' (Williams 1962; Ball 1990a), schools needed to promote attitudes and skills appropriate for a late twentieth-century advanced economy. Neo-conservatives, on the other hand, wanted schools to promote the traditional values of respect for the family, private property and authority. And neo-liberals believed that managers and teachers needed to behave in more entrepreneurial, consumer-satisfying ways. These same currents of thought continue to be influential within the New Labour government, although these have been fused with concerns about social justice in the formulation of a so-called third way. As we shall see later in the book, New Labour's 'pragmatic eclecticism', with its attempt to combine neo-liberal, conservative and more humanistic social democratic values in the formulation of educational policies, is fraught with tension.

Analysing post-welfarism in education: beyond school effectiveness and indeterminacy

At the time of planning the research upon which this book is based, two important collections of papers had begun to draw attention to the values dimensions of the market and associated modes of management (Keat and Abercrombie 1991 and Heelas and Morris 1992). In one of these collections, Raymond Plant had warned that the application of private-sector principles to public-sector services may constitute a threat to 'civic responsibility' and result in 'the erosion of social values in favour of private and self-interested ones' (1992: 89); and that 'in the state sector the introduction of markets, quasi-markets and the dominance of contract might well deprive us of ethical principles such as service and vocation, which are essential to the efficient delivery of services' (1992: 94). Plant also saw the market as a potential threat to one of the basic principles underpinning public-sector provision; 'the idea of respect for persons: that people themselves should not be treated as commodities, or as means to the ends of others' (1992: 92). In a similar vein, Stewart and Ranson (1988) had sought to demonstrate how the values inherent in business management practices are sometimes at odds with those necessary for the effective provision of public services. Most obviously, there may be a conflict between concerns related to making a profit and those related to meeting social needs. And writing in 1984, Maw *et al.* had drawn attention to the threat which a business culture may constitute to 'notions of professionalism and professional autonomy, the caring and welfare-oriented aspects of education's role, and education's purpose in promoting social equity' (Maw *et al.* 1984).

However, whilst there had been much *speculation* about the cultural implications and value effects of post-welfarism in education (see also Ranson 1990 and Raab 1991) there had been little empirical and empirically-based theoretical work in this area. The emphasis in research into the reform of schools had been – and continues to be – primarily on the structural and technical aspects of the new system (for example, Levacic 1995 on the local management of schools (LMS), Glatter *et al.* 1997 on the responsiveness of schools and Fitz *et al.* 1993 on the autonomy available to headteachers and senior management teams); or on the outcomes of change for specific constituencies (for example, Lee 1992a and 1992b on special needs, Troyna *et al.* 1993 on ethnic minorities and Deem *et al.* 1995 on governors). However, it remains the case that little sustained attention has been given by researchers to values, to institutional languages and cultures, to changes in decision making practices and the social relations of school-ing, or to the relationship between these elements (although there are notable exceptions – see, in particular, Grace 1995, Menter *et al.* 1997 and Woods *et al.* 1997). It is these substantive gaps in the research that this book is intended to fill.

Furthermore, individual studies have tended to focus on particular initiatives, such as LMS, changes in school governance and the national curriculum. However, these policies combine and interact in complex ways and so should not be researched in isolation. This book, therefore, takes a more holistic perspective than is typical in the literature and looks at the compound effects of post-welfarist policies on schools.

The approach adopted in this book is mainly a response to concerns about two major – and very different – influences within recent educa-tional research: that of post-modernism and what I refer to as the *celebration of indeterminacy*, on the one hand, and the school effective-ness and improvement industry, on the other. My concerns about these trends are underpinned and informed by a commitment to the trans-formation of educational practice as a contribution to a politics of social justice. I would suggest that policy research can contribute to such a project in two ways: first, by exposing the various forms of injustice and oppression which education policies can generate and, second, by identifying spaces within which socially just pedagogies, practices and policies are emerging or can emerge. I want to suggest that the two currents I outline below hinder both of these projects and that an alternative analytical approach is needed.

The celebration of indeterminacy is an analytical trend that places a great deal of emphasis on complexity, ad hocery, messiness and unpre-dictability. It is informed by *particular variants* of post-modernist theory. The approach is typified by Richard Bowe, Stephen Ball and Anne Gold's *Reforming Education and Changing Schools* (1992), a case study of the early impact on secondary schools of certain aspects of the 1988 Education Reform Act – more specifically, the national curriculum and local management of schools. 'The policy process', they argue, 'is one of complexity, it is one of policy-making and remak-ing. It is often difficult, if not impossible to control or predict the effects of policy, or to be clear about what those effects are, what they mean when they happen' (Bowe *et al.* 1992: 23). This perspective seems to have been quite influential on other policy researchers in education. Halpin and Fitz (1990), for instance, explicitly endorse their concept-ualisation of policy implementation, as do Penney and Evans (1992), Raab (1994) and Crump (1997). The celebration of indeterminacy, it would seem, is becoming an orthodoxy amongst education policy analysts.

The optimism of this approach, achieved through the emphasis it places on the capacity of subjects to contest and rework dominant discursive frames has great appeal. And I agree with Bowe *et al.* and the other celebrants of indeterminacy, that the process of policy implementation is messy, complex, ad hoc and results in unintended and unforeseen outcomes. This is because those who produce policy texts have never been able to control precisely how they are interpreted and put into practice on the ground. However, I want to argue that it is possible to overstate the messiness, complexity and ad hocery associated with policy implementation. This kind of conceptualisation can obscure patterns of domination and oppression which, I argue in this book, are being exacerbated by recent policy developments.

The conceptualisation of implementation employed by Bowe *et al.* draws on a particular approach to discourse theory which 'interprets discourse as a site and object of struggle where different groups strive for hegemony and the production of meaning and ideology' (Best and Kellner 1991). The following extracts from Bowe *et al.* illustrate their approach:

> We would want to approach legislation as but one aspect of a continual process in which the loci of power are constantly shifting as the various resources implicit and explicit in texts are recontextualized and employed in the struggle to maintain or change views of schooling . . . This leads us to approach policy as a discourse, constituted of possibilities and impossibilities . . . While the construction of the policy text may well involve different parties and processes to the 'implementing' process, the opportunity for re-forming and re-interpreting the text mean policy formation does not end with the legislative 'moment'.
>
> (Bowe *et al.* 1992: 13)

> [P]olicy is not simply received and implemented within [the context of practice] rather it is subject to interpretation and then 're-created' . . . Practitioners do not confront policy texts as naive readers, they come with histories, with experience, with values and purposes of their own, they have vested interests in the meaning of policy. Policies will be interpreted differently as the histories, experiences, values, purposes and interests which make up any arena differ. The simple point is that policy writers cannot control the meanings of their texts. Parts of texts will be rejected, selected

out, ignored, deliberately misunderstood, responses may be frivolous etc. . . . we must not see power in relation to policy as a fixed dimension. In patterns of contestation claims to power will always be tested in the process, power is an outcome.

(Bowe *et al.* 1992: 22)

It is our contention that it is in the micro-political processes of the schools that we begin to see not only the limitations and possibilities State policy places upon schools but, equally, the limits and possibilities practitioners place upon the capacity of the State to reach into the daily lives of schools.

(Bowe *et al.* 1992: 85)

Bowe *et al.* are not textual or discourse 'reductionists', that is they do not believe that it is possible to reduce everything to discourse or textuality. And they note that 'interpretations are not infinite' and that 'different material consequences derive from different interpretations in action'. But they only note this in passing and go on to reiterate their main point that 'the meanings of texts are rarely unequivocal. Novel or creative readings can sometimes bring their own rewards. New possibilities can arise when 'national' policies intersect with local initiatives' (1992: 23). They argue that whilst 'some teachers may be oppressed by the National Curriculum text . . . we find considerable evidence of creative responses' (1992: 96).

I do not disagree with any of these statements. What I am objecting to is the degree of emphasis. So much emphasis is placed on the interpretability of texts, the unpredictability of policy outcomes, the complexity of the policy process, the ability of individuals working in schools to respond creatively to state policies, that broad patterns of oppression and domination generated by those policies and associated discourses are obscured. Bowe *et al.* appear to be tacitly adopting a Foucauldian conception of power, as fragmented, fluid and always open to contestation:

Power's condition of possibility . . . must not be sought in the primary existence of a central point, in a unique source of sovereignty from which secondary and descendent forms would emanate; it is the moving substrate of force relations which, by virtue of their inequality, constantly engender states of power, but the latter are always local and unstable. The omnipresence of power: not because it has the privilege of consolidating everything under its invincible unity, but because it is produced from one moment to the next, at every point or rather in every relation from one point to another. Power is everywhere; not because it embraces everything, but because it comes from everywhere.

(Foucault 1990: 93)

[A]s soon as there is a power relation, there is a possibility of resistance. We can never be ensnared by power: we can always modify its grip in determinate conditions and according to precise strategy.

(Foucault 1988: 123)

And they are open to the same criticisms that have been made about Foucault's work, initially by Poulantzas (1978), that overt and violent forms of state oppression and class dominance are understated. These criticisms are summarised nicely by Best and Kellner (1991):

Foucault rarely analyses the important role of macro-powers such as the state or capital. While in *Madness and Civilisation* and *Discipline and Punish* he occasionally points to the determining power of capitalism, and in *The History of Sexuality* he sees the state as an important component of 'biopower', macrological forces are seriously undertheorised in his work. In Foucault's defence, it could be argued that his intention is to offer novel perspectives on power as a diffuse, disciplinary force, but his microperspectives nevertheless need to be more adequately conjoined with macroperspectives that are necessary to illuminate a wide range of contemporary issues and problems such as state power (as manifested in oppressive laws or increasingly powerful surveillance technologies) and the persistence of class domination and the hegemony of capital.

As Poulantzas (1978) observes, Foucault seriously understates the continued importance of violence and overt repression. For Poulantzas, by contrast, '*State-monopolised physical violence permanently underlies the techniques of power and mechanisms of consent: it is inscribed in the web of disciplinary and ideological devices; and even when not directly exercised, it shapes the materiality of the social body upon which domination is brought to bear*' (1978: 81). Poulantzas does not deny the validity of Foucault's perspective of disciplinary power, he only insists that it wrongly abstracts from state power and repression which, for Poulantzas, are the conditions of possibility of disciplinary society.

(Best and Kellner 1991: 71–2)

My point is that Bowe *et al.* emphasise 'the limits and possibilities practitioners place upon the capacity of the state to reach into the daily lives of schools' at the expense of exposing the way in which state policies and dominant discourses impose a highly constraining disciplinary framework on schools and local school systems. The material and ideological consequences of that disciplinary framework, I will argue, include an increased subjugation of teachers, a closer alignment of schooling with capitalist values and the exacerbation of inequalities of provision along class lines.

The celebration-of-indeterminacy approach to research is not only diversionary, it also carries with it the potential to function in a legitimatory way. Post-welfarist reforms are justified by their proponents partly on the grounds that they are more democratic, that they are effecting a decentralisation of power: headteachers and governors are being empowered, we are told, at the expense of out-of-touch and overly-bureaucratic local authorities, and parents are being empowered in relation to schools and local authorities. I am concerned that research which overemphasises the diffusion of power inadvertently reinforces and supports neo-liberal versions of the market, which, as I shall argue in subsequent chapters, are simply not supported by the evidence.

An emphasis on macro-structures is discouraged not only by postmodernist trends within the academy but also (for very different reasons) the school effectiveness and improvement lobby, and it is to this current in educational research to which I now want to turn.

School effectiveness and improvement research is a large and growing industry that is essentially atheoretical. The research is concerned primarily with 'problem solving'. In other words, it takes:

> the world as it finds it, with the prevailing social and power relationships and the institutions into which they are organised, as the given framework for action. The general aim of problem-solving is to make these relationships and institutions work smoothly by dealing effectively with particular sources of trouble.
>
> (Cox 1980: 129)

This is what C. Wright Mills called the *bureaucratic ethos*. 'Research for bureaucratic ends', he wrote, 'serves to make authority more effective and more efficient by providing information of use to authoritative planners' (Mills 1959: 117). On the whole, the effectiveness/ improvement research tends to ignore or at least oversimplify the socio-economic context within which schools operate. So-called effective schools are said to have specific characteristics which are believed to be primarily, if not wholly, controllable by school-based agents of change. In other words, it is usually assumed that a good school manager with a strong team of teachers will be able to create 'effective schools' and 'effective classrooms' regardless of the structural or material conditions within which they are operating. Similarly, the 'new' school management literature (e.g., Caldwell and Spinks 1988, 1992) encourages school managers not to concern themselves with those things which are beyond their control, namely the socio-economic or policy context, 'but to get on and do the job by focusing on their own little domain of the school' (Angus 1994). Gerald Grace (1997) has observed that there are writers in the school improvement tradition who do acknowledge the importance of the socio-economic context, usually in introductory chapters. However, this tends to be done in a tokenistic fashion and any apparent appreciation of the significance of context tends not to be integrated into the rest of the analysis (see, for example, Stoll and Fink 1996).

An oversimplified conception of the relationship between socio-economic context and teachers' practices is also a notable feature of New Labour's education policy. Under the influence of educational advisors who are rooted within the school effectiveness and improvement industry, New Labour has argued that it is time education policy focused less on structures and more on the processes of teaching and learning. For example, the Labour Party's education policy document, *Excellence for Everyone: Labour's Crusade to Raise Standards*, published in December 1995, concluded: 'For too long in Britain we have got the balance wrong in our education system. We have had a concentration on structures, when we need to concentrate on getting the content right' (Labour Party 1995: 34). A similar argument was made by Michael Barber in *The Learning Game* (1996) – a book endorsed on its front and back covers by Tony Blair. In that book, Barber – who was later appointed as first head of the DfEE's (Department for Education and Employment) Standards and Effectiveness Unit established by New Labour in 1997 – derided and caricatured concerns about the relationship between education, policy and the economy. Barber suggested that arguments about the structural causes of educational failure divert attention from where much of the responsibility for educational failure actually lies – the schools, their managers and their teachers. A similar perspective is apparent in much of the recent high-profile media coverage of cases of 'failing' schools. These reports have, on the whole, neglected to consider the extent to which 'failing' schools 'fail' because they are disadvantaged by a punitive funding structure and because they exist within hierarchically ordered and effectively selective local systems of schooling.[2] Instead they have focused on 'weak' management and 'poor' teaching. Nor does there appear to be much recognition in public debates around schooling that the discourses of post-welfarist education policy, like markets, target setting, performance monitoring and inspection, are not neutral mechanisms for 'improving' schools. In particular, there seems to be little appreciation that these discourses have embedded within them a set of values about what education is, and is for, and that they function as powerful disciplinary mechanisms for transforming manager and teacher subjectivities and the culture and values of schooling.

I am making what should be the somewhat obvious point here that managers, teachers and schools do not operate in a vacuum, as so much of the school improvement, policy and media rhetoric implies. The content and form of schooling is, and always has been, heavily influenced by such things as the mechanisms by which resources and students are distributed to schools and to classrooms within schools, the examinations system, and the physical and social space of the school and the classroom, as well as by the management styles and practices of headteachers. Such factors are in turn shaped, to a significant degree, by the socio-economic, policy and discursive contexts within which the school system operates. Hence, I would want to

2 An exception was a high-profile and very detailed series of articles by the journalist Nick Davies (1999a, b and c) that appeared on the front pages of *The Guardian* on three consecutive days in September 1999. Using the example of two Sheffield schools, Davies graphically illustrated how the education market exacerbated inequality and polarisation in education (on the basis of class and race) and the extreme challenges faced by schools serving socio-economically distressed communities. The articles prompted a reply by David Blunkett, Secretary of State for Education at the time, in which he reiterated New Labour's view that, in order to solve the problem of failing schools, the main emphasis must be on better management. 'A good head' he wrote 'makes a big difference regardless of where a school is located. A strong, dynamic headteacher is vital to success – so is a committed team of teachers with high expectations of what can be achieved.' Whilst Blunkett stressed the importance of additional money in the article, he also attempted to disparage those who express concern about structural inequality. Those who draw attention to the problems arising from inequality and segregation in the schools system were accused of 'political correctness' and of having low expectations of poor children. 'In tomorrow's Britain,' Blunkett wrote, 'we cannot afford to write off any child, just because our schools system doesn't fit neatly into preconceived notions of political correctness – whether they be of the right or left' (Blunkett 1999: 21).

argue that any adequate understanding of schooling and teachers' work necessarily involves a serious consideration of the influences of the wider contexts within which schools are located.

My central concern in this book is to do precisely what the school effectiveness research and post-modernist accounts of the kind described above do not do. That is, I will explore the ways in which the socio-economic, policy and discursive environments within which schools operate are shaping the culture and values of schooling. In doing so, I will demonstrate how the PWEPC functions as a powerful disciplinary mechanism of re-acculturation and how processes of re-acculturation appear to be generating various forms of oppression and injustice, including the reproduction and exacerbation of entrenched socio-economic inequalities, the subjugation of teachers, a closer alignment of schooling with the values of capitalist society, and a move towards more traditional and socially regressive pedagogies. I will also explore the contradictions and tensions at work within the post-welfarist education system.

However, in rejecting the celebration of indeterminacy approach, I do not want to dismiss every aspect of post-modernist theory. Indeed, there is much to be gained from taking on board post-modernist emphases on diversity, complexity, contestation and the contingent and on micro-level relationships, processes and practices. But such insights need to be combined with a neo-Marxist emphasis on structure. As Apple has argued:

> It has proven all too easy in educational scholarship and theory to accept Foucault's epistemological position whole and uncritically. There is a world of difference . . . between emphasizing the local, the contingent and non-correspondence and ignoring any determinacy or any structural relationships among practices. Too often important questions surrounding the state and social formation are simply evacuated and the difficult problem of simultaneously thinking about both the specificity of different practices and the forms of articulated unity they constitute is presumed out of existence as if nothing existed in structured ways . . . In my mind it is exactly this issue of simultaneity, of thinking neo and post together, of actively enabling the tensions within and among them to help form our research, that will solidify previous understandings, avoid the loss of collective memory of the gains that have been made, and generate new insights and new actions.
>
> (Apple 1996a: 141)

This book takes seriously the issue of *simultaneity* that Apple is drawing attention to here. Thus, neo-Marxist state-centred forms of analysis are used to explore the dynamics of policy change and it is suggested that post-welfarist policies have some *generalised*, structuring effects across the school system which are producing various forms of injustice and oppression. At the same time, however, local variations in the internal regimes of control in schools are recognised, the influence and inter-weaving of social, economic and biographical factors are acknowledged, and I deploy a 'rich' conception of social justice that looks beyond narrow Marxist class-centred conceptions and draws on insights from feminist, anti-racist and post-modernist theory and practice.

Part I

Post-welfarism and the reconstruction of English schooling

2 Learning to lead: headteachers and the new managerialism

This first part of the book is concerned with exploring the kinds of schools that post-welfarism is producing. More specifically, it uses ethnographic material to examine how the language, values and processes of schooling are changing as a consequence of post-welfarist policies and discourses, and it seeks to reveal something of the complexities of these shifts. Since headteachers play such a crucial role in shaping school responses to the post-welfarist education reform project, Part I begins in this chapter with an analysis of the changing practices and orientations of school headship.

The PWEPC has constructed a new role for headteachers that is characterised by shifts in focus, style, practices and language. Since 1988 headteachers have been responsible for their school's budget and for ensuring that it is managed efficiently and cost-effectively. They now have to make decisions about the appointment, utilisation and dismissal of staff and the purchase and use of physical resources. And they have to try and win the hearts and minds of their staff in order to manage the conflict and dissent produced by the PWEPC (Gewirtz et al. 1995). All of these tasks have demanded a change in the style and practices of headship. In effect, they have required a new mode of coordination in schools (see Chapter 1). Unpredictable and changing budgets create a sense of urgency and uncertainty, which in turn constitute pressures for the decisive assertion of the managerial prerogative.

The growing significance of headship – or what is increasingly being called leadership – is highlighted and reinforced by the proliferation of education management texts and courses, and by the growing influence of school management gurus on educational policy and practice. Brian Caldwell and Jim Spinks, for example, the Australian authors of the best-selling publications, *The Self-Managing School* (1988) and *Leading the Self-Managing School* (1992), have acted as policy consultants in

England and New Zealand as well as Australia (Whitty *et al.* 1998). They emphasise the importance of what they call 'transformational leadership' in the creation of self-managing schools. And, as Whitty *et al.* (1998: 53) have commented, their 'exhortations to engage in goal setting, policy making, planning, financial budgeting, implementing and evaluation performance are more reminiscent of business [norms than of those] previously associated with educational institutions.' Gerald Grace (1993) has reported on the far-reaching impact that such texts are having on schools and other educational institutions. 'Not only do texts on various aspects of education management begin to be a significant sector of educational publishing but, more pervasively,' he writes, 'the language, assumptions and ideology of management begin to dominate the language, consciousness, action and modes of analysis of those working within the education sector' (1993: 353). In a similar vein, Stephen Ball has written of the reverential place that the term 'management' now holds in education circles:

> The need for 'good' management in schools, colleges, and universities provides a point of massive agreement among educational practitioners of all leanings and persuasions. Management is firmly established as 'the one best way' to run educational organisations. Management training is becoming de rigeur for anyone who aspires to high office in educational institutions. The unchallengeable position of management effectively renders discussion of other possibilities for organisation mute.
>
> (Ball 1990b: 153)

But what does the pre-eminence of managerial approaches to school headship mean in practice? What has changed in the ways that school headteachers think and talk about their role? These are the questions I want to address in this chapter. My approach is to focus on the case of one inner-city comprehensive school, Beatrice Webb.[3] The school is an interesting case because what happens there, and the way its staff and governors talk about what happens, brings into sharp focus the discursive shift that appears to be evident on a larger scale in the management

---

3 The school is one of four London secondary schools researched in some depth as part of the study, 'Schools, Cultures and Values', funded by the UK Economic and Social Research Council. This chapter draws on interview and observational data gathered over a two-year period of fieldwork in the school (from 1994 to 1996). All names have been changed to protect the anonymity of the school and participants in the study. See Appendix for details of the research methods used.

of the English public sector as a whole, and within the public sectors of a number of advanced capitalist states. Within the recent sociological literature on organisational change in education and other welfare sectors, this shift has been conceptualised in various ways. Angus (1994) describes a move away from participative/professional forms of administration to technical/managerial ones. Grace (1995) contends that a social democratic phase of school headship has been superseded by a market phase. Others have argued that the market may be facilitating an assertion of a 'technical rationality' in school management over and against a 'substantive rationality' (Bottery 1992).[4] Yeatman (1993) describes how the culture and influence of 'humanistic intellectuals' have been replaced by those of 'the technical intelligentsia'. Clarke and Newman (1992a and 1992b, 1997) suggest that the restructuring of the welfare state by the New Right represents an attack on 'bureau-professionalism' and an attempt to replace it with a 'new managerial regime'. Storey (1992) writes of an increased emphasis upon 'individual' as opposed to 'collective' relations with employees. This emphasis is manifested in the utilisation of more direct forms of communication and involvement, in integrated reward systems and in the linking of remuneration to performance rather than to a 'rate for the job' (Storey 1992: 14). Such shifts in management strategies have in part been facilitated by periods of high unemployment and by legislation aimed at weakening trade unionism.

Although the concepts used in these various formulations are different, essentially they denote overlapping clusters of characteristics. My intention here is to explore in detail the ways in which the kind of discursive shift denoted by such broad conceptualisations is being played out within the context of a single inner-city comprehensive school. But before turning to the case of Beatrice Webb, I want first to delineate two ideal-type discourses of school headship – 'welfarism' and 'new managerialism'. I am using the term welfarism to represent the organisational mode of coordination, leadership style and values associated with the welfarist settlement. 'New managerialism' refers to the mode of coordination, leadership style and values associated with post-welfarism. My intention is for these types – which incorporate

---

4 The emphasis of technical rationality is upon the development of techniques, procedures and organisational practices that are intended to facilitate speed of decision making, coordination, the setting and reviewing of objectives, good financial controls and information, cost improvement, responsiveness and consumer loyalty. The emphasis of substantive rationality is upon the intrinsic qualities of the 'product-process' – here education, teaching and learning (Considine 1988).

the conceptualisations listed above – to function as heuristic devices and as starting points for an examination of the shifting and complex positioning of real people and institutions acting out their roles in specific places and over specific periods of time. The discourses are, of course, not all-embracing. There are other discourses of headship which are neither welfarist nor new managerialist. My decision to concentrate on the shift from welfarism to new managerialism, however, is based on the contention that it encompasses some of the most common transitions in the languages and practices of headship.

So what is the cluster of characteristics which comprise welfarism? First, welfarist provision is characterised by a particular mode of coordination, that is, a particular 'articulation of modes of power which connect the structures, cultures, relationships and processes of organisational forms in specific configurations' (Clarke and Newman 1992a: 5). Clarke and Newman refer to this mode of coordination as bureau professionalism which embodied 'the Fabian archetype of expertise coupled with the systematic organisation of services through the regulatory principles of administrative categories' (Clarke and Newman 1992a: 4–5). As Newman explains:

> Bureaucratic administration was a rational, rule bound and hierarchical approach to co-ordinating complex systems of people and resource processing. Bureaucratic administration provided the organizational context in which welfare professionals – doctors, teachers, social workers etc. – exercised their professional judgement. This combination of administrative rationality and professional expertise guaranteed the 'neutrality' of the welfare state and protected the exercise of professional judgement in the delivery of social welfare.
>
> (Newman 1998: 335)

But welfarism denotes more than a particular mode of coordination or organisational form. It also encompasses a *style* of headship (or a way of managing) and particular beliefs about the *ends* and purposes of headship; that is, both method and substance (although, as we shall see, the two are not necessarily aligned in practice).

For analytical purposes I will make a clear but heuristic separation between welfarist and managerialist headship. The archetypal welfarist headteacher operates according to a substantive, as opposed to a technical, rationality and belongs to Yeatman's category of the 'humanistic intellectual', that is he or she is:

not at all indifferent to theoretical and analytical debates concerning strategies of redistribution and social justice, and the so-called crisis of the welfare state ... The welfarist headteacher is a 'public servant' who is 'clearly committed to a conception of a public interest, which is not reducible to a sum of private preferences'.

(Yeatman 1993: 348)

However, welfarism is a 'broad church' that draws on diverse and often contradictory sets of concepts. It embraces a whole range of values and practices, and there are stark differences of opinion over what constitutes the public interest and which strategies are most appropriate for serving it. For example, comprehensivism in England, a key condensate of identification and commitment within educational welfarism, has a history of distinct 'liberal' and radical interpretations. Moreover, dominant notions of what constitutes good welfare practice and hegemonic constructions of who are the subjects of welfare and what their needs are *have shifted over time* and have always been contested (Langan 1998; Saraga 1998). Amongst the most popular welfarist discourses in education since the late 1960s have been those which revolve around ideological commitments to: equality of opportunity; valuing all children equally; equal and supportive relationships; caringness; child-centredness; comprehensive schooling; assimilationism; multi-culturalism; anti-racism; girl friendliness; anti-sexism; developing critical citizens; democratic participation and social transformation. In addition, 'collegiality, service, professionalism and fair-dealing are valued' (Clarke and Newman 1992a: 17).

The work of the new manager may well not be informed by any of the 'old' welfare values which characterised much educational thinking and practice in the 1960s, 1970s and early 1980s. The new managerialist headteacher is likely, although not necessarily, to be a recent recruit to a position of senior management with little or no experience of educational management prior to the 1988 reforms. (There has been a concomitant exodus of pre-reform headteachers via early retirements of various kinds.) Whilst welfarist managers tend to be socialised within the field and values of the particular welfare sector they are working in, new managers are more likely to be generically socialised within the field and values of 'management':

In contrast to welfarism, new managerialism views bureaucratic control systems as unwieldy, counterproductive and repressive of the 'enterprising spirit' of all employees. Its notion of the route to competitive success is to loosen formal systems of control . . . and to stress instead the value of motivating people to produce 'quality' and strive for 'excellence' themselves. Managers become leaders, rather than controllers, providing the visions and inspirations which generate a collective or corporate commitment to 'being the best'.

(Newman and Clarke 1994: 15)

For the new manager in education, good management involves the smooth and efficient implementation of aims set outside the school, within constraints also set outside the school. It is not the job of the new manager to question or criticise these aims and constraints. The new management discourse in education emphasises the instrumental purposes of schooling – raising standards and performance as measured by examination results, levels of attendance and school leaver destinations – and is frequently articulated within a lexicon of enterprise, excellence, quality and effectiveness. The main characteristics of the two discourses are summarised in Table 2.

Table 2 Main characteristics of welfarism and new managerialism

Welfarism	*New managerialism*
Public-service ethos	Customer-oriented ethos
Decisions driven by commitment to 'professional standards' and values, e.g., equity, care, social justice	Decisions instrumentalist and driven by efficiency, cost-effectiveness, search for competitive edge
Emphasis on collective relations with employees – through trade unions	Emphasis on individual relations – through marginalisation of trade unions and new management techniques, e.g., Total Quality Management (TQM), Human Resource Management (HRM)
Consultative	Authoritarian/'macho'
Substantive rationality	Technical rationality
Cooperation	Competition
Managers socialised within field and values of specific welfare sector, e.g., education, health, social work	Managers generically socialised, i.e., within field and values of 'management'

Having outlined the clusters of characteristics which comprise these ideal types of headship, I now want to focus on the case of Beatrice Webb, in order to explore in some depth the content of the kinds of discursive shifts identified by Clarke and Newman, Angus, Grace and Yeatman, as they occur at an institutional level. In doing so, I will introduce some messiness into the apparently neat polarisation of these binaries. I should stress, however, that space restrictions prevent me from portraying accurately the *details* of events within the school, which means that at times I employ thumbnail sketches of what in practice are more complex phenomena.

Beatrice Webb School

Public sector markets are supposed to operate on Darwinian principles. Strong institutions, defined as those which attract custom and maximise income, are meant to thrive; the weak, 'the unpopular', are meant to go to the wall. In terms of the market, Beatrice Webb is a weak institution. Heavily undersubscribed, it has around 500 pupils although there is room in the school for almost double that number.[5] Only a handful of the students who attend do so because they choose to go to Beatrice Webb. The majority are there for one of the following reasons: they have failed to get in anywhere else; they have been excluded from other schools; or they belong to refugee or homeless families which have been placed in temporary accommodation near the school. As a result, Beatrice Webb has a highly transient population. Each week the staff bulletin lists departing and new students. There are usually at least four or five students in each of these categories. Sixty per cent of the students speak English as an additional language and approximately 35 per cent are refugees. There are children from Turkey, Cyprus, Bangladesh, Kurdistan, Somalia, Eritrea, Ethiopia, Vietnam, South America and Sri Lanka. In September 1995 the local authority administered a reading test to all Year 7 (first-year secondary) students in the authority. Of these eleven year olds at Beatrice Webb, 32 per cent were diagnosed as having a reading age of less than seven. Less than 8 per cent of the year group had a reading age which was at or above the average for their chronological age.

5 A note on my use of tense: In general, throughout the book, background descriptions of the schools are written in the present tense to indicate clearly that not only the schools but the issues and agenda around new managerialism are ongoing. However, where I am writing specifically about data collected some time ago, I indicate this by using the past tense.

In 1996, 9 per cent of students gained five or more GCSEs grades A–C, compared with the national average of 45 per cent. Many of the families of students at the school have contact with the social services and a high proportion of students is characterised as having learning or emotional and behavioural difficulties.

The school building looks neglected. Poor recruitment (and therefore a small budget) means there is not enough money to replace cracked windows or to repaint the shabby interiors of the three buildings which make up the school. The curriculum is heavily under-resourced. There are very few textbooks and there is a heavy reliance on work-sheets. Students are not allowed to write on the worksheets or take them out of the classroom because departments cannot afford to photocopy more. Instead, the children have to spend lesson time copying the worksheets out by hand. During the 1995–6 school year the art department had just £1.50 to spend on each child. The head of art was interviewed half way through the school year, by which time she had run out of pencils, was low on paper and the paintbrushes were falling apart. One of the consequences of the paucity of resources in art is that it is relatively difficult for students at Beatrice Webb to demonstrate the range of artistic skills and approaches necessary to gain a good GCSE grade.[6] Similar accounts of lack of resources and the educational implications of that lack were elicited about other areas of the curriculum in the school.

Beatrice Webb was one of four schools researched as part of a study looking at the impact of marketisation and associated reforms on school cultures and values. The schools were selected in order to high-light contrasting features in terms of 'market position', responses to the market, socio-cultural differences in the composition of student and governing bodies, differences in the history and constitution of management teams, and in institutional 'visions' and mission statements. Beatrice Webb was chosen because of its inner-city location and characteristics, its poor market position and the apparently strong welfarist orientation of the headteacher. We were interested to find out what was happening within schools whose culture and values were, at face value, at odds with the hegemonic discourses of management and the market. Six months into the project the welfarist headteacher, Susannah English, resigned and was replaced by a new head, Brian Jones, who displayed many of the characteristics of the new manageri-

---

6 Although despite this, the school's results in art are above the national average (see Chapter 5).

alist headteacher outlined above. This chance event in the research presented us with the opportunity to compare the two headteachers.

Ms English

Susannah English referred to herself as 'a leftover from the romantic Sixties'. A former history teacher who had always worked in inner-city schools, she became head of Beatrice Webb in 1989. Ms English's educational philosophy and priorities were represented by the published school aims (which were developed before she joined the school and have since been changed by her successor). The first four aims were as follows:

(a) At Beatrice Webb we aim to work with parents and others to help students with their personal and social development, and to acquire, enjoy and use the knowledge and skills to understand and explore their world and the means of changing it.
(b) We aim to provide a wide range of learning experiences and opportunities through a broad and balanced curriculum and through all aspects of school life in order to meet the needs and abilities of all students.
(c) We aim to create a rigorous, challenging and creative environment in which our students can achieve high educational standards and leave school with the desire and ability to become life-long learners.
(d) We aim to welcome people into the school, encourage respect for other peoples, their values, cultures and rights, including their right to learn.

For Ms English, the primary aims of the school were to foster personal and social development, to encourage children to look at the world with a critical eye, with a view to making it a better place, and to ensure that the needs and abilities of all children were met. She was also concerned that the children achieved high educational standards but her rationale for this was not the instrumental one of meeting the needs of the economy or of enabling individual students to get jobs when they leave school. Her central rationale was to develop the motivation of children to learn and to enable them to become 'life-long learners'. Ms English was committed to the strand of welfarism which views education as being important 'for its own sake' and as a tool of social transformation.

Significantly, the theme of relationships and a whole set of concepts related to that theme were central to the way Ms English talked about the school and her role as headteacher. For example, in describing the positive things about the school, she focused (perhaps idealistically) on the relationship between teachers and students:

> A lot of the teachers . . . seem to really like both the challenge and the actuality of working in a place like this where the children are so responsive . . . and the relationships with the children are extremely warm.

She was also fascinated by 'the power struggles and the . . . relationships . . . adult to adult, adult to children, children to children'.

In addition, gender relationships and gender dynamics were of vital interest to Ms English. She was somewhat concerned about the gender imbalance amongst students in the lower school. She was much more concerned about the gender imbalance amongst the senior staff and about the cultural implications of that for the way the school operated as an organisation:

> The staff is heavily male and I am now the only senior member of staff who is a woman . . . which is a great sadness to me. By senior, I mean I'm the only one in the Senior Management Team now. We've lost the deputy head recently, who was both female and black, which was really sad . . . And the main grade teachers tend to be more women than men – slightly . . . – so we've got an imbalance here in gender for staff, which I mind about a great deal. I think it actually affects things. It's a very male-dominated staff. All kinds of things get affected by that – the way people argue and discuss and try and put pressure on them and so on.

Ms English was committed in principle, she claimed, to consultative and non-hierarchical modes of management. However, she believed that LMS[7] did not allow for the operation of what she viewed as these essentially *feminine* modes of management:

> I think LMS has changed how people can manage schools and I think that links directly to the gender thing. I'm not saying all women managers have a – what I would call a more feminine style of management – they don't obviously – but it's much more

---

7 Established by the 1988 Education Reform Act, LMS devolved responsibility for the management of school budgets and the appointment and dismissal of staff from the local authority to schools.

difficult under LMS, and if you are a woman, to be . . . open and consultative and less hierarchical. It's much more difficult than it used to be. And all those important decisions about money and people's jobs and so on – it's really hard. And it's the kind of thing that a lot of women don't want to go into management to deal with . . .[8] The sort of archetypal headteacher that people have got in their mind when they want to sell their school is a man, and he's white and he's probably got a grey suit on, probably hasn't got a beard any more . . . but . . . I've seen these people come through the ranks anyway, and now I think it would be interesting to see whether the new appointees to headships will continue to be women . . . The [decisions] on staffing are really difficult to be consultative and open and democratic [about] . . . We're in financial difficulty at the moment, and dealing with that . . . it is very difficult indeed. [It would] be nice to say, 'Let's all look at this, it's all our problem, let's look at how we all share it and resolve it'. In the end, the reality is it's not going to be that people will chip in and say, 'Okay, I'll go, I can see it's for the good of everybody'. That isn't how it happens. Somebody's got to be making clear decisions based on good educational principles, and that can be done by a group of people and can be consulted on, but in the end, the carrying through is going to have to be done by a group of fairly hard-nosed people.

Some degree of compromise or contradiction may already be evident in these comments and I would suggest that the practice of headship is in part defined by such compromises. Nonetheless, in aligning herself with a set of values and practices focused on the quality of relationships, democratic modes of management and the personal and social development of children, Ms English distanced herself *rhetorically* from the business values and practices of the new managerialism. In practice, however, she did tend to act in an authoritarian manner with teachers. For example, towards the end of her headship she attempted to impose a new faculty structure on the staff, despite the bitter opposition of all but a handful of teachers. Heads of department

8 Previous research (Gewirtz *et al.* 1995) and case study work in another school in this project suggest that such an essentialist relationship between gender, values and leadership style is analytically untenable. And, to confuse the picture further, Clarke and Newman (1997) argue that 'new management' in fact involves a 'feminisation' of management with a stress on 'the skills of communication and culture building, network and partnership management, providing good relationships with customers and workforce, and managing complex processes of change and transition' (1997: 73).

were asked to apply for the new faculty head's posts but they boycotted the process. Only two out of the twelve heads of department broke ranks and applied for the new posts. However, Ms English's authoritarianism in this and other instances cannot be explained solely in terms of the pressures of devolved management but also has to be seen in the context of the peculiar institutional dynamics of the school.

Ms English was somewhat disdainful about the pedagogical beliefs and practices of a significant body of her staff. Although politically militant, these mainly male teachers of working-class origin tended to be educationally conservative and trenchant in their opposition to any changes in their working practices. Because Ms English did not value them as teachers and because of the reluctance of this influential group of staff to cooperate with any of her suggestions for change, she tended to make decisions in what all of the teachers we interviewed saw as a high-handed manner. Thus, it would be too simplistic to argue that marketisation imposed on Ms English an authoritarian management style. It would appear that at Beatrice Webb, market pressures may well have combined with pre-existing micro-political tensions to reinforce an approach to management which was already somewhat 'macho' (i.e., assertive and confrontational), despite Ms English's claimed preference for more feminine styles of headship.

Even so, Ms English was also resistant to the 'Chief Executive' aspects of the new headteacher's role – responsibilities for managing finances and the school buildings, appointing and dismissing staff, and marketing the school. Her focus of interest lay in classroom practice and the curriculum, sometimes described as the 'leading professional role', and she was 'uncomfortable' with the substance and implications of a primary focus on budgetary concerns. She displayed exactly what Clarke and Newman (1992a: 10–11) describe as 'a complex sense of dislocation and uncertainty about the possibilities and prospects of becoming a new manager combined with a sense of confusion and loss about old certainties'. She was resistant to the idea of becoming a bilingual speaker of the old and new management idioms:

> I do know about working in the classroom and I do know about working with children, and I know quite a lot about the curriculum. Now all of that – the curriculum in particular – has been removed; not how you teach, but what you teach, that decision has been removed. And instead I've been handed huge decisions like . . . sorting out the roofs, or reglazing, or hiring and firing staff . . . And I still resent it, that's the . . . Luddite in me. I want

to go back to somebody else making all those decisions because they're so uncomfortable.

In practice, Ms English, to a certain degree, tacitly accepted these new tasks and responsibilities. However, her reluctance in doing so arguably marred her capacity to perform them effectively, where effectiveness is defined as maximising the school's income and its market position. For example, Ms English's antipathy towards tasks related to finance seemed to have affected her ability to ensure that the school was getting the most it could from the LEA because it would appear that, although primarily funding is worked out according to the published LEA formula, there nevertheless remains a degree of LEA discretion in precisely how the formula is interpreted and applied. There is some room for financially astute headteachers and governors to pressurise LEAs to give them more money. This privileges those schools with the more financially literate headteachers. Ms English did not appear to be one of these:

Interviewer: So what's happened with finance under LMS?
Ms English: I couldn't – I'm not good enough at finances to sort of give you an off the cuff figure. And I don't know that [the LEA] ever told us; I know they were supposed to by law, how much it cost us but . . . all I know is that it's been difficult ever since we've been here; and that's partly been – and it's been in [the authority's] interest, the education officers . . . and some of the members, to fudge it.

Furthermore, where some schools created specialist financial posts at senior management level, Beatrice Webb resisted this trend on principle and, as Ms English acknowledged, the school may have suffered financially as a result:

Ms English: We've resisted in our Senior Management Team [having] the man who walks around with computer printouts . . . with all those sort of figures and you ask a question and, you know, paper flies and calculators come out. We don't have somebody like that and we wouldn't want it because that's not the way we want to work, but I suppose the advantage of that is then they're the kind of people who can respond to . . . consultation and say what it will mean for the school.

Interviewer: Why is it that [you've resisted] having them?

Ms English: Oh well partly it's a gender issue. It's not the main thing, but there is a gender issue that it's always the men who get in charge of the money . . . And I see that happening in schools and I think that's a quick route, it's . . . like an accelerated route to headship and I very much resent that as a kind of stereotyping that does happen. And it's a bit the same with women being in charge of girls . . . and uniforms, that kind of thing, it's . . . the reverse thing you have, and it's the hard face . . . it's what modern education is all about is being able to manage the finance. But also we wanted as a Senior Management Team . . . to share those kinds of decisions and the understanding of it between us.

Here, old and new languages and concomitant institutional practices are in direct opposition; expedience is set against principle.

Another example of how Ms English's reluctance to embrace the values and practices of the market may have affected the school's income and market position stems from her principled stance on marketing. Ms English had gone some way to improve the school's marketing practices. She was in regular contact with the headteachers of the school's feeder primaries, she produced a glossy brochure and in 1992 she appointed a new deputy headteacher whose principal role was to improve recruitment to the school. However, Ms English drew the line at trying to attract more middle-class parents by 'massaging the image of the school':

Ms English: Ultimately if we don't get the children, that's tough on us, but our obligation is to the children we do have; that's our first obligation, to educate those children to the best that we can so that they get the best out of the school . . . Now I come into quite a lot of conflict with the education officers and members because they want the school to be more balanced. They say, 'your job would be easier if you didn't have quite so many time-consuming demands on the school [from] refugee children or less able children and so on', which is quite true, 'so you ought to invest a lot of your energies and time into recruiting better'. And I'm saying 'no', because our very first obligation is to those children. We have a bit of a difference about that.

Interviewer: Are they saying that the kind of children you have is giving you a bad image?

Ms English: I think it's true, I think it's true. And I think . . . parents who do the choosing and send children some distance, who tend to be the middle-class parents, aren't going to choose a school where they see 60 per cent of the children speak English as a second language, because they'll believe that that will bring down the quality of what goes on in the classroom for their little darling. Or you could . . . even . . . put a more racist interpretation on it. They don't want to be in a school where there are a lot of black faces or Asian faces because they will see that as being 'black equals rough, and Asian, well some of them are hard working but some of them need bilingual support or English as a second language support'. I do think it operates like that . . . and the difficulty in judging how you present that is how far you're prepared to go along with it, and I think that's one of the weaknesses of local management and this whole money-following-pupils business. It does lead you into temptation about uniform, and massaging the image rather than the reality, so that you get the nice glossy brochures, the pictures of boys all in uniforms sitting in assembly looking angelic and Christian and white. Whereas that's not the reality of this school and I'm not prepared to package it in a way that implies that, either by putting people in uniform or putting black kids out of sight when we do our publicity shots. But I think the price to pay for that is quite high [because] then you're not going to be selected, and that's quite a difficult tension all the time. Sometimes I think people would like to see the back of me, because it might be easier not to have somebody saying those kinds of things. And I suspect, when I go, uniform will be introduced.

It was this unwillingness to compromise such anti-racist and egalitarian educational values in the face of market pressures that made Ms English essentially a welfarist, and she was clearly aware that her values and principles did not fit easily within the prevailing values and expectations of school headship.

Six months after I first interviewed her, Ms English resigned from her post. Her reasons were partly to do with the micro-politics of the school. Her relaxed approach to discipline, her tendency, as many teachers perceived it, to take the side of the pupils against the teachers, her gender and, possibly, her upper-middle-class background consistently provoked a hostile and recalcitrant approach from a male dominated, politically militant and educationally conservative staff. These factors, together perhaps with a failure to communicate her ideas and decisions effectively, made it difficult for Ms English to achieve all that she wanted in the school and left her frustrated and over-stressed. But the frustration and stress were not simply products of internal relations within the school. The tensions and hostility between the head and her staff were clearly exacerbated by the disjuncture between the head's welfarist commitments and the values and practices generated by the new policy environment. The socio-economic and linguistic make-up of Beatrice Webb's student population and its mobility, meant that the school was heavily penalised financially by the education market. This was translated into heavy debts, drastic underfunding of the curriculum, insufficient language and learning support, a shabby, demoralising physical environment and fears of redundancy amongst staff. Adequate funding would not have guaranteed the school's success. Nor, in all likelihood, would it have healed the rifts between staff and the headteacher. But it would have removed the fear of redundancy and it would have improved working conditions and thus may have reduced tensions, leaving the Head in a stronger position to put her commitments into practice. Ms English was replaced by Mr Jones.

Mr Jones

Mr Jones 'knew' what he had to do to make Beatrice Webb 'successful', as success is defined by the market/management discourse, and he was prepared to do it. He displayed few uncertainties about what he hoped to achieve at Beatrice Webb or how he would achieve it and at times he presented the 'visionary' qualities of the new manager, linking leadership with passion. Mr Jones saw his primary task as balancing the budget, which was £43,000 in deficit. At the time of his appointment, the school employed 38 'FTEs' (full-time equivalents) but there was only enough money in the budget for 29. Balancing the budget involved making cuts, for example, by cutting off-site PE provision, making redundancies and abolishing the 'referral room' (otherwise known as the 'sin bin'), where 'disruptive' children were meant to go when they were sent out of lessons. The referral room was staffed by senior managers and was, therefore, expensive, although there were believed to be good educational as well as financial reasons for its abolition.

Making cuts involved doing things Mr Jones felt personally uncomfortable with but which he saw as necessary in management terms.
The difference between Mr Jones and Ms English on this score was
exemplified by his decision to enforce retirement on a teacher who
had taught in the school for many years and was considered by both
Ms English and Mr Jones to be good. Retaining him did not make
'financial sense' and Ms English's decision to keep him on was, according
to Mr Jones, an example of 'inappropriate compassion'.

Mr Jones' other strategy for balancing the budget was to increase the
school roll, with a particular emphasis on attracting more middle-class
students. As he told the deputies at a senior management meeting:

> All the school effectiveness research shows that only seven per cent
> of student achievement is down to what the school does. Most can
> be explained in terms of the characteristics of the students coming
> to the school. So we need to make sure that we attract more able
> students.

> (Observation notes)

In order to attract more 'able' students, Mr Jones introduced a uniform. His argument was that not only does a uniform create an image
of discipline and is, therefore, attractive to the 'aspirant classes' but
also that it inculcates a more serious attitude towards school and
school work. So, here market and educational rationales were elided
(see also Ball 1998). In addition, Mr Jones intended to rewrite the existing school aims, cited above, because they emphasised the 'wrong'
things. He told the staff on his first day:

> In schools we care but we need to express our deep caring through
> providing a learning environment and opportunities for work, so
> we need to take one step back from the indulgence of trying to
> solve all the students' problems. They have different backgrounds
> but this is not a branch of the social services, and we are not social
> workers. Although we have to educate with a knowledge of
> students' backgrounds we need to put work and education at the
> top of the agenda.

> (Observation notes)

In effect, Mr Jones wished to narrow the focus of the concerns of
the school to concentrate more exclusively on teaching and learning.
In doing so, he intended to make the school more instrumentally

oriented and performance focused. This would, in turn, couple the schools' primary concerns more directly with the performance indicators established by the government, which are partly intended to provide 'choosers' with 'relevant' market information.

Mr Jones' initial plans included the refurbishment of the foyer and his own office. During my first meeting with him, he took me into his office and said:

> Look at this room, it's down at heel like the rest of the school. We need to give the right impression to middle-class parents who we need to attract if the school is to be saved. It should look more like a chief executive's office. I'm getting rid of these shabby old filing cabinets and getting three spanking new ones and I'm replacing those tables with a round table and comfortable chairs to sit round for meetings. And he wasn't going to use recycled paper like the old head which, he said, was very admirable in environmental terms but hardly gave the right image.
>
> (Observation notes)

As with the other headteachers we researched, Mr Jones was very concerned with the semiological subtleties of image, symbols and presentation (Gewirtz *et al.* 1995). In fact, by the end of his first year in the post, he had relocated his office to a place which was less accessible to students, staff and parents, creating a formal 'chief executive' style suite consisting of an office with adjoining meeting room. Free access to the head's 'suite' was limited to those who knew the code that opened the self-locking door – the head, his secretary and his two deputies. This was in stark contrast to Ms English's informal, cosy, slightly chaotic, usually open-doored room, which was frequently visited by students. Part of Mr Jones' rationale for reorganising space in this way was to distance himself from the day-to-day activities of the school in order to release time and mental space for strategic planning issues. The shift from 'leading professional' to 'professional manager/ chief executive' is clearly signalled in this. This physical reorganisation of space is highly symbolic of the gap that has opened up in values, purpose and perspective between senior staff with a primary concern with balancing the budget, recruitment, public relations and impression management, and teaching staff with a primary concern with curriculum coverage, classroom control, student needs and record keeping (Bowe *et al.* 1992; Pollard *et al.* 1994; Gewirtz *et al.* 1995; McHugh and McMullan 1995).

In making these changes, Mr Jones had to try and bring the staff with him. His visionary work was part of this. However, he had to pay particular attention to the small but vocal group of staff who successfully blocked a number of the initiatives that the previous headteacher had tried to introduce and who were characterised by the senior management team as 'dinosaurs'. Getting the support of this group of staff involved Mr Jones in attempts to establish his working-class credibility. For example, at the first meeting with staff he talked about his background of being brought up in an over-spill council estate. It also involved engaging in male-bonding activities, for example, playing football and making jokes about filo-fax size. None of these tactics were available to Ms English. In addition, Mr Jones made a point of telling the staff what a good job they had been doing (even when he did not really believe it) in order to bolster their morale and win their support. This is a classic tactic of 'people-centred' new management – 'The new manager must be attentive to the potential contribution of everyone in the organisation and create a climate in which they feel their contributions will be valued and welcome' (Clarke and Newman 1992b: 3). Mr Jones was also keen on the use of what he liked to refer to as Machiavellian management techniques. For example, in senior management meetings he regularly expressed a concern to make decisions appear curriculum driven when they were essentially budget driven. Another strategy he used was to decide, in advance of consultation, small 'concessions' he was prepared to concede to staff, to manufacture the appearance of genuine negotiation.

Mr Jones was able to speak about the school using very different lexicons and registers, for example, in senior management team meetings as opposed to staff meetings. He was 'multilingual' in the sense that he could move relatively easily between the 'older' language of public service (which has embedded within it a language of equal opportunities) and a number of new languages of school management – the language of the market (public relations, entrepreneurship, marketing and recruitment), the language of financial management (the budget, plant management, income generation), the language of organisational management (corporate culture, human resources, quality, effectiveness and performance) and, when required, the new language of curriculum (programmes of study, units, modules, levels of attainment, national testing). In effect, these languages marked out a series of overlapping 'cognitive communities' (Douglas 1987) of people working with shared meanings acquired through a series of communicative exchanges. One of Mr Jones' skills was his capacity to translate between these languages and move across the cognitive communities in which they were embedded. This involved an ability to argue that market driven, financial or managerial decisions were compatible and indeed could enhance good educational practice.

But Mr Jones' use of different languages was not *just* a tactic. In a number of senses, he continued to be influenced by welfarist discourses. Mr Jones believed that balancing the budget would contribute to the well being of the students by enabling him to channel money into improving language support and resourcing the curriculum. Mr Jones had spent most of his career in inner-city schools and he appeared genuinely committed to providing a good education for working-class young people. The new management systems he introduced, for example, meetings with a predefined purpose, followed up by action and the monitoring of that action, were intended ultimately to contribute to the improvement of curriculum planning and classroom practice. And, like Ms English, Mr Jones was increasingly concerned about the gender imbalance of the senior management team and relationships in the school, relationships amongst staff and between teachers and students.

Conclusions

The two discourses identified in this chapter – welfarism and new managerialism – represent two largely opposed conceptions of the nature and purposes of schooling and they also relate to more general visions of the nature of society and citizenship. In real terms, the *pure* forms of these discourses are probably hard, but not impossible, to find. However, the beginnings of a discursive shift were discernible at Beatrice Webb even over the short time-scale of the research, with the appointment of the new headteacher functioning as the dramatic catalyst. The new head brought with him not just new ways of speaking but ways of thinking and acting which differed markedly from the previous Head, and which had potentially significant material consequences for teachers and students and school life more generally. For the new ways of speaking described, justified and helped to implement budgetary cuts, workforce restructuring and new decision-making structures, which reduced opportunities for debate.

There is no doubt that benefits may be accrued from the task-centredness of new management. At Beatrice Webb ossified and ineffective practices were challenged and loosened-up. However, within the prevailing incentive structure and its performance-related funding mechanisms, the logics of new management also suggested a reorientation of the school was to be attempted, away from its primary emphasis on the immediate needs of its current community to 'improvement' by intake manipulation, whereby highly valued clients were to be sought out at the expense of the 'needy'. For Mr Jones recognised that there was no financially viable role in the educational market for an institution like Beatrice Webb, as it existed under the headship of Ms English. With its intake as it then was constituted, it could not compete within the funding regime put in place by the 1988 Education Reform Act: its students were undervalued, they were costly, and to all intents and purposes the school could not be expected to achieve at the *absolute levels* of neighbouring schools.

What I have tried to convey in this chapter is the fact that the market revolution is not just a change of structure and incentives. It is a transformational process that brings into play a new set of values and a new moral environment. In the process it generates new subjectivities. The role and sense of identity and purpose of school managers are being reworked and redefined. In this way, new managerialism functions as a 'relay' (du Gay 1996: 66) for the implementation and dissemination of the post-welfarist project. As I argued in Chapter 1, it provides a means by which school practices can be realigned to performance criteria set by the state.

However, I want to emphasise that there is no simple or absolute process of change at work. This chapter has focused on discourses of headship – on the way in which headteachers talk and think about and act out their roles – but I have also exemplified the links, and some of the dissonances, between the languages and practices of headship. And, of course, these discourses do not go uncontested. Whilst both Ms English's welfarism and Mr Jones' new managerialism were embraced enthusiastically by some members of staff, they were also challenged and resisted from within the school. However, under Mr Jones' 'transformative leadership', the establishment of new decision-making structures and the relocation of the head's office significantly reduced opportunities for overtly challenging new managerial policies and practices. Indeed, they were designed with just this purpose in mind. It has not been the purpose of this chapter to explore these struggles over language, policy and practice, but their importance needs to be acknowledged.

What I have been able to show, by focusing on the individual headteachers, is that the new languages of enterprise, quality and excellence grate against existing and embedded welfarist languages but may still encompass aspects of the welfarist project, even if the possibilities for the realisation of the project are altered significantly. Headteachers bring with them into this transformation personal qualities, complex histories and social positionings which mean that a straightforward totalising fit within a dominant discourse is unlikely. For example, Ms English's welfarism is intermingled with an apparent elitism in that her warm and mutually respectful relations with students do not extend to her relationships with staff, a number of whom complained that she treated them in a dismissive way. At the same time, Mr Jones' energetic new managerialism appears to be underlain by a genuine commitment to working-class youth. Thus, social positionings, like gender and social class, can interrupt or inflect the acting out of dominant discourses.

The changes in languages and practices that are embedded in and brought about by the replacement of one dominant discourse (welfarism) by another (managerialism) are mediated and inflected by a set of 'local' structural, institutional and individual factors. These factors are the market position of the institution within the local competitive arena, the micropolitics of the institution, and the professional histories and biographies of key players within the institution. The headteacher is the most important of these, as the main 'carrier' (and literal embodiment) of, or impediment to, discursive reworking.

3 Ethics and ethos
Conflicting values in the managerial school

In Chapter 2, I described the marketisation of education as a trans-formational process, associated with which is a shift in values and the emergence of a new moral environment. However, I also suggested that this is not a simple process. The shift in values and language associated with marketisation – and the construction of the post-welfarist settlement more generally – is contested and struggled over. In trying to respond to the pressures created by the market, headteachers and teachers find themselves enmeshed in value conflicts and ethical dilemmas, as they are forced to rethink long-held commitments. It is such conflicts and dilemmas that are the focus of this chapter. The issues surrounding them will be explored through a consideration of the experiences of one school, Northwark Park,[9] at a critical 'moment' of its 'adaptation' to the new post-welfarist policy environment. Like Beatrice Webb, discussed in the previous chapter, North-wark Park found itself in the early 1990s having to confront the issue of institutional survival in a marketised context.

Ethical dilemmas and value conflicts arise because the market functions as a system of rewards and punishments, a disciplinary framework, fostering particular cultural forms and socio-psychological dispositions and marginalising others. Within a market culture it is acceptable for there to be winners and losers, access to resources which is differentiated but unrelated to need, hierarchy, exclusivity, selectivity and for producers to utilise whatever tactics they can get

9 Northwark Park was one of 14 schools where fieldwork was conducted between 1990 and 1993 as part of the ESRC-funded study 'The operation and effects of markets in education'. As in the previous chapter, pseudonyms are used to protect the anonymity of the school and those who took part in the research. See Appendix for details of the research methods used.

away with to increase their market share and to maximise profits. In short, there is pressure on individuals (both producers and consumers) to be motivated first and foremost by self interest. That self interest may be institutional – when it is activated in relation to the acquisition of institutional rewards (e.g. of the school); or it may be individual – when it is activated in relation to personal rewards (e.g. of the parent, child or teacher). The social psychology of the market discourages the universalism and collectivism that in theory underpinned 'comprehensivism' – one of the principle ideological and organisational components of welfarism from the 1970s onwards. There is, of course, considerable contestation around what precisely comprises the comprehensive ideal and around how, or indeed, whether that ideal can be realised, given the practical difficulties associated with reconciling the principle of universalism with a system of schooling which recognises and engages appropriately with difference and diversity. Nevertheless, one of the key assumptions of comprehensivism was that the educational needs of all children in an area, regardless of class, 'race', gender or ability, should and could be met by the local neighbourhood school. This principle is threatened not just by choice and competition but also by the controls that have been placed on the market. The national curriculum, testing at four key stages, the publication of those test results in the form of league tables and the emphasis on target setting and performance monitoring within a context of underfunding represent potentially powerful mechanisms for influencing the way schools function in the market place. For example, the publication of league tables acts as an incentive for schools to select students (where they are able) on the basis of ability. Funding shortages provide an additional incentive to select – 'less able' children and children for whom English is a second language, for instance, are more expensive to educate than 'more able' children who are proficient in English. Funding constraints also threaten other aspects of certain versions of comprehensivism because adequate mixed-ability teaching and the integration of children with special needs are expensive ways of organising learning.

The extent to which an individual school is able to resist the culture of the market depends largely on its market position. A heavily oversubscribed school is least likely to face a situation in which it needs to change what it is already doing in order to attract pupils. Where schools are unsuccessful in market terms (i.e., they are undersubscribed) the potential for resistance is lowest and market-induced ethical dilemmas are therefore most pronounced. This was the case with Northwark Park.

Northwark Park

In the early 1990s Northwark Park was undersubscribed and under pressure. An ex-Inner London Education Authority (ILEA) school, it is located on the eastern edge of Northwark where it abuts the neighbouring authority, Streetley. It takes about one third of its children from primary schools in that authority. The school's intake is predominantly working-class, although there is a small core of white middle-class children, described by staff in the school as having liberal/left-wing parents who choose the school because it is local, comprehensive and non-uniform, 'and a lot of them have been involved in Labour Party politics, educational and housing issues, that kind of thing and basically believe very much [in] a local authority' (headteacher).

Approximately 45 per cent of the children are white, 45 per cent are African-Caribbean and the remaining 10 per cent is made up of children from other minority ethnic groups, including children with a South Asian background and African, Chinese and East European students. The school's poor market position could well have something to do with its relatively short and rocky history. It was opened in 1986 as an amalgamation of two schools, one of which itself was the product of an earlier amalgamation. In 1991 the school was one of four in the authority threatened with closure. Although it won its campaign to stay open, the uncertainty surrounding its possible closure was harmful in terms of recruitment. Northwark Park also suffered from a reputation of being 'tough' because, as the headteacher put it: 'each time it got going as a mixed school, they amalgamated it with a boys school. Therefore it has fought actually the image of a boys' school for quite some time'. And its location near to Broughton tube station and Broughton High Street, and adjacent to a pub with a history of drug activity, were other factors beyond the control of the school which were seen to be affecting its reputation.

However, the impression one gets from spending time in the school is actually very different from its rough, tough, macho reputation. The school building is small and carpeted, and the atmosphere is calm, quiet and relaxed. The following comment by one of the NAS/UWT (National Association of Schoolmasters/Union of Women Teachers) representatives is typical of how the school was described by its teachers and confirms this impression: 'the school has always been a very friendly school. It's not the sort of school that you feel much physical intimidation . . . students are very friendly, staff are very friendly'.

Northwark Park had a stable and experienced staff but, therefore, also an expensive staff which led to speculation amongst some teachers that senior management might, in the context of formula funding, be forced to make redundancies:

> The school is losing money because they have such experienced staff, so there is always the thought that if you can get rid of some of the experienced staff and bring in some young probationers, it would actually be saving the school some money, so do you sacrifice experience for financial reasons?
>
> (Acting deputy head)

An expensive staff means less money for other (non-human) resources, like books: 'We barely have enough really to replace damaged books these days' (maths teacher). Undersubscription compounds the funding shortages. Whilst money is in short supply in the school, the needs of many of the children are great. Like Beatrice Webb (see Chapter 2) and many other inner-city schools, Northwark Park has a relatively high turnover of children: 'we had a lot of first generation immigrants coming into the area, so we tend to take those obviously, because we're a school that's got vacancies, so they tend to get pushed here, and then you get a lot of families who will settle for a year or so and then move out, so we lose a lot of children' (head of Year 7). The intake of the school is skewed towards 'lower ability' children[10] and the school-based Education Welfare Officer (EWO) has contact with a high proportion of the children in the school. When I interviewed the EWO she had just over 100 open cases in a school with less than 700 on roll, not counting those children she worked with on a casual basis. She estimated that 'a sixth probably of the school . . . sometime or another is referred'. She attributed this high proportion to the reputa-

---

10 In order to try and ensure an even spread of ability throughout their schools, the ILEA employed a system of banding. Children were tested in the last year of primary school and allocated to one of three 'ability bands' with pupils of the highest measured ability being put in band one and those with the lowest in band three. The theory, although not the practice, was that each ILEA secondary school should have an ability spread which reflected the ability spread in the ILEA school population as a whole. In 1992 Northwark Park had the second lowest intake of band one children in the LEA and the highest proportion of band three children. By 1999, owing to the introduction of selection (by this time Northwark Park had become a selective specialist school), the proportion of band one children had increased but the top two bands nevertheless continued to be under-represented in the school.

tion the school has as a caring school and the selective nature of another local school:

> It's known as a small caring school and a school that's known as caring, I think, gets a high proportion of children with problems and because Hutton, which is our nearest secondary school in Northwark, has always had a much higher profile, so they have always been in the position where they can pick and choose a lot more.

The education welfare service within the authority as a whole was cut in the early 1990s and, since amalgamation in 1986, the special needs department at Northwark Park had also been progressively reduced in size:

> As our staffing has shrunk and shrunk . . . from about five full timers down to two full timers, it's basically down to the basics of English and Maths, and some Science if we can, not all classes get it . . . We're an easier area to cut obviously than others because we're not an area of the curriculum, as such.
>
> (Head of special needs)

An additional effect of cuts had been an increase in class sizes in certain subjects and the use of teachers to teach subjects they have not been trained to teach in:

> Now in this school it is not recognised that practical subjects require smaller classes . . . We've got people who usually teach art and come in here to do odd periods which is very – well they've got no commitment to the department, they show no interest in the department, so basically it drags the department down.
>
> (Technology teacher)

Thus, the combination of a high level of need amongst the children, cuts in special needs provision and in particular curriculum areas, undersubscription, *per capita* funding and a parsimonious local authority meant that the school's resources were extremely stretched. Northwark Park was a school fighting for its survival. If it ignored the market, it died. Given its undersubscription and its overall funding position, the school had little option but to take competition for students very seriously: 'The system is now changing, which means

Table 3 Mismatch between comprehensive and market values

Comprehensive values	Market values
Student needs	Student performance
Universalism	Differentiation
Mixed-ability	Setting
Cooperation with other schools	Competition with other schools
Resource emphasis on 'less able'/special educational needs (SEN)	Resource emphasis on 'more able'
Caring ethos	Academic ethos
Led by agenda of social/educational concerns	Led by agenda of image/budgetary concerns
Oriented to serving needs of local community	Oriented to attracting 'motivated' parents
Integrationist	Exclusivist
Emphasis on good relationships as basis of school discipline	Emphasis on extrinsic indicators of discipline–like uniform
Distinctive	Emulative

we . . . cannot stay as we were. We will have to perform in some way in order to survive' (teacher governor).

However, the need to change in response to new conditions threw up ethical dilemmas. The school's staff and governors had been ardently committed to a particular set of ideals which they associated with comprehensive education, but they believed that the new market structure of educational provision was not conducive to the retention of a comprehensive culture (see Table 3). There was, therefore, a significant mismatch between the ideological commitments of the teachers and the culture of the market, and the starkness of this dichotomy produced dilemmas in the school's response.

The educational culture of Northwark Park was very much part of the ILEA culture where:

> every school had to have an equal opportunities statement, and were encouraged to actually pay particular respect to girls, to black children, and to children with disabilities, including statemented children.

> (Chair of governors)

Northwark Park was committed to the integration of children with special needs and, as we have already seen, it had a reputation for being a caring school. The staff had been particularly concerned to promote equal opportunities for girls: some all-boys groups had been introduced 'so that girls' experience of the classroom would not be that they were swamped' (headteacher) and times were set aside when only girls could use the library.[11] Another crucial element that characterised Northwark Park's particular version of comprehensivism was its policy on mixed-ability teaching, whereby all lessons in all subjects and years were taught in mixed-ability classes. The other elements that were part of the comprehensive school culture of Northwark Park included a commitment to cooperation with other local schools, a relaxed and friendly atmosphere in the school, good relationships between students and staff, and no uniform.

Clearly, I would be presenting too romantic a view if I were to portray Northwark Park pre-Education Reform Act as a kind of model comprehensive school. Whilst the staff expressed a commitment to a set of values which they associated with the comprehensive school, it would be naive not to question the relationship between rhetoric and practice, and the school was not without its internal critics. There was a general concern expressed by a number of members of staff, including the new headteacher, Barbara Swallow, that the school had traditionally failed to challenge children academically:

> I think in the past there were schools [and she is clearly implying that Northwark Park was one of these] weren't there, that saw its image as a caring school and there was always a kind of sub text to that, which meant a not very high achieving school.
>
> (Headteacher)

> We do get on reasonably well with the students . . . but a lot of Northwark Park is that we don't challenge, as a staff we don't challenge, and I think that's been one of our failings in the past.
>
> (Head of Year 7)

---

11 The issue of equal opportunity policies in relation to gender is perhaps one example of compatibility between comprehensive and market values. Since one of the concerns of Northwark Park's management is that the school is unpopular because of its macho image, policies designed to promote gender equality would seem to be a good marketing strategy in this particular instance.

The chair of governors, in particular, was concerned about what he believed to be low expectations of working-class children in general and black boys in particular in the school:

> There are issues like the performance of black boys in an area where there isn't work for black youths . . . it's the boys who very much get the worst out of the school, and out of the job market.
>
> [The Head's] view is that the staff have almost sort of a corporate profile about what they think they're about, which needs to be budged. Firstly, they think they're there to help the underprivileged working-class kids, and to that extent they resent the high-flying kids from middle-class homes who come and seem to do well in the school . . . and I think she thinks that their attitude to both is wrong, that they need a far more systematic and less condescending approach to the bulk of the kids who come to the school.
>
> (Chair of governors)

Similar doubts about opportunities for black children to perform well in the school were voiced by one of the parent governors. There was also a concern that the school alienated black and Asian parents who were reluctant to become involved in the school: 'we haven't got very many black staff here so at a parents' evening, if a black parent does come to a parents' evening, they'll only see a couple of Asians, two Asian teachers and one black teacher, out of . . . 49 staff. So the school is very white, the senior management is totally white, it's nearly all male' (teacher governor).

Like many comprehensive schools then, there would seem to have been at Northwark Park a gap between comprehensive values and comprehensive practice within the school. But the gap was acknowledged, particularly by certain governors, including the Chair, and apparently by the head too. What I want to address here are particular aspects of the conflict between the desire to narrow this gap and the need to survive in the local education market place.

The staff were *reluctantly implicated* in the market. They did not like it, but they were part of it and most recognised the need to respond to it:

> I don't think you can have a premise that you have winners and losers in education. I don't think society can afford to run on those sorts of principles . . . and I think this sort of, this market

place business is potentially very dangerous. I mean we have to respond to it, that's the problem, that's why we're sort of running round in circles at the moment, because we can't just take the moral high ground and say, we will have nothing to do with that, we have to be part and parcel of it.

(Deputy head)

I don't believe in parental choice at all. I think really parents should send their children to the local school. I don't believe in private education either. But it's there and it's staying so we have to make the best.

(Head of sixth form)

But how did they deal with this *reluctant implication*, how did they 'make the best' of it? Ideally they wanted to adhere to their principles, to what they saw as the comprehensive ethos of the school, whilst becoming more successful in the market place. It was a fragile balance and there were varying degrees of sacrifice which the staff and governors were prepared to make. It is possible to visualise a *values spectrum* along which individuals drift (Gewirtz *et al.* 1995). On one end of the spectrum are those who are reluctant to change, resistant to abandoning any of their principles. The governing body of the school had on it a majority of left-wing members who were strongly opposed to any values drift. The chair of governors, Dan Kennedy, for instance, had been active in socialist education politics for many years. An ex-ILEA sub-committee chair, he was also a governor of a secondary school in Streetley, a past vice-chair of governors at Streetley College and Secretary of the Streetley Socialist Education Association. As we have already seen, Dan Kennedy was particularly concerned about what he believed to be low expectations of black and working-class children by teachers at Northwark Park. The governors were seen as constituting the school's ethical conscience:

I think the governors, our governors, are quite political and, by and large, they are former ILEA governors, so they are, I mean they are political, they are left-wing, by and large, and I don't think for one moment they approve of the sort of market place philosophy in education, and I think it just is taking them some time and will take them some time, to come to terms with what it implies.

(Deputy head)

The head believed that some governors would just give up, rather than compromise their values: 'I think there are some who will probably just stop being governors, because they hate the situation so much.' Some of the staff shared the governors' opposition to abandoning what they saw as key elements of the school's comprehensive culture:

> it is a pretty friendly school where the children are on the whole fairly pleasant to each other, and to other people, not very confrontational, possibly a little bit too laid back, and we don't really want to change that, except for the laid back attitude. We don't see ourselves as being sort of a grammar school in another guise, we don't see ourselves, we don't want to become a new secondary modern. We would like to continue to be the community secondary school.
>
> (Head of sixth form)

However, the headteacher had drifted further along the values spectrum, arguing that the community school is incompatible with a competitive structure of provision:

> I think that it's the kind of school, with the kind of staff and governors, who would like to see, the governors would certainly like to see a community school, and I think it's taking a lot of people quite a long time to think themselves into . . . the different situation, that the '90s are not like the '70s . . . and the community school is not going to happen with LMS and with GM[12] schools and we have to take on the competition, whether we like it or not.
>
> (Headteacher)

Like Mr Jones at Beatrice Webb (see Chapter 2), the headteacher, Barbara Swallow, was able to move relatively easily between the language of the market and the older language of public service. And whilst the headteacher was prepared to use the language of competition

12 Under the 1988 Education Reform Act schools could 'opt out' of local authority control and choose to be funded directly by central government. These grant-maintained (GM) schools were better funded then LEA schools, had more autonomy and controlled their admissions. The grant-maintained sector has since been abolished by the 1998 School Standards and Framework Act. However, the status differentials which the GM schools policy produced have not been eradicated, since the 1998 Act has allowed schools which were previously GM to retain a separate status from other LEA schools (by calling themselves 'foundation' schools).

and engage with the market, she still wanted to hang on to aspects of comprehensivism but without the community part. The elements she wanted to adhere to were a broad curriculum, a comprehensive intake, and equal opportunities policies for gender and 'race'.

John Fox, the deputy head cited earlier, would seem to have been located even further along the values spectrum towards a more ready acceptance of participation in the marketplace. He appeared to be toying with the idea of a shift towards a more grammar school-type ethos to enable the school to sell itself more effectively. He described – admiringly it would appear – changes that had occurred in the nearby opted-out girls school, Martineau:

> I'm not saying it's lost its comprehensive ideals, but Kath Davies, who is the head there, in my view has set herself up as near as damn it to a traditional girls' grammar school . . . I mean it's obviously attracted a lot of people. You know, you can imagine trying to put that across here and I think you might run into difficulties.

Presumably, the difficulties he was talking about relate, at least in part, to the reluctance of governors and many of the teachers in the school to compromise their comprehensivist principles.

The market sets the kind of values which are associated with comprehensivism against institutional survival and thus against jobs and livelihoods: the market, as a disciplinary framework, fosters the social psychology of self-interest (both institutional and individual) which, in many respects, conflicts with the collectivist, universalistic psychology conducive to a system of provision informed by comprehensive values. In the rest of the chapter, I want to look at five key issues around which conflicts arose in the school out of the clash between comprehensive and market values, between attempts to retain elements of a culture of collectivism and the social psychology of self interest.

Expanding the intake

All of the conflicts I want to look at emanated from the pressure on Northwark Park to expand its intake. The new local structure of provision involved schools opting out, informal selection and fears that Northwark Park would become a sink school:

> I fear that what will happen is that Hutton, which is a mixed school, and that Martineau, which is a girls' school, will grow and grow and grow in strength . . . and what will happen is then

we will go back to being a secondary modern school.

(Head of Year 7)

What we are determined is that we will not become the [sink] school in the authority, to put all the kids who have been chucked out of grant-maintained schools . . . my aim is to get us full.

(Headteacher)

There was a general recognition that the school must attract a more diverse clientele. But there seemed to be different conceptions of what particular sections of the community the school should be targeting. The head commented that, 'I'm not saying we're looking for middle-class parents . . . but we're looking for motivated parents'. Yet, elsewhere in the interview, her concern did seem to be for the school to appeal to middle-class parents. The head also talked about the possibility of beginning to attract South Asian children: 'I think that we have not tried very hard to get into the Asian community. It's an area we ought to do some more work on'. John Fox, the deputy head, expressed a desire to attract the newly affluent working-class or lower middle-class parents:

We always have had, and still do have, a nucleus of what I suppose you would call sort of very middle-class, very sort of politically aware parents, who consciously send their kids here because they like certain aspects of the school, but what we miss out on is the other sort of, a lot of that sort of middle band of people who have, you know, real sort of aspirations for themselves and for their children as well. I don't know what you'd call them . . . like electricians and plumbers and people like that who are enjoying a certain sort of affluence, you now. They tend to avoid us and I'm not sure why that is.

And Dan Kennedy, the chair of governors, saw potential for the school to appeal to black parents from Streetley, dissatisfied with what's on offer there:

The temptation for Northwark Park is to capitalise . . . on the fact that it really is very close to the border of Streetley, and . . . Streetley inherited a situation where it has 50 per cent of its secondary aged kids being exported, I mean the figures that I had at the end of the ILEA, you are more likely to find band one children moving . . . there is an option, a planning option, which is that Northwark Park could establish itself doing well by black kids, for example.

Cutting across these varied (but not necessarily incompatible) views of who the school should be targeting and how the public is segmented were conflicting rationales for the expansion. It was at this juncture that comprehensive values began to vie with market-induced values. Kennedy's strategy for expanding the intake by making the school attractive to black parents from Streetley was clearly consistent with his concern that the school should be more responsive to the needs of black children. The attempt to attract more 'motivated' parents was defended by other members of staff as being essential if the school was to remain comprehensive. A comprehensive school, it was argued, is dependent on there being a 'balanced' or comprehensive intake:

> If you can attract a good range of intake, if you're full, and with-out, still within the comprehensive ideal, have a range of ability, rather than being weighted at the bottom, then I suppose by and large all the students benefit from that sort of balance.
>
> (Deputy head)

> I think what people here would say is that every school should take its share of problem families, problem children, children with special educational needs, we don't want those children at all, but a school which is full of children like that, very easily becomes a sink school, because nobody puts the resources in that you need to deal – that's why secondary modern schools didn't work.
>
> (Headteacher)

Yet there is a fine line between wanting to expand one's intake in order for it to remain comprehensive and wanting to expand it in order for it to become selective. Dan Kennedy suggested that Martineau, the nearby grant-maintained school had already crossed that line: 'I think you'll find that you get so much double talk about what people think they're doing or what they say they're doing . . . I mean the opting out schools say they're opting out in order to preserve comprehensive education'. What Kennedy was hinting at here was that some schools, whilst claiming they wanted to remain compre-hensive, were in fact selecting on the basis of motivation. They were, in other words, adopting the kinds of informal admissions policies used by some of the voluntary-aided ILEA schools and more formally by City Technology Colleges and other specialist schools. Whilst Kennedy's comments were directed at Martineau, in some of the comments made by staff at Northwark Park, it was already possible to detect an ambiguity on the question of selection. Alongside arguments about a balanced intake being necessary if the school was going to continue to function as a comprehensive, were arguments that hinted at a desire to be selective or to somehow gain in status within the local economy of schooling: 'Ideally every school wants to be over-subscribed, so it does have some control over who comes in . . . to be in a position to say, no' (acting deputy head).

By 1998 the school had succumbed to the pressure generated by the selective practices of other local schools, which had meant that Northwark Park's intake had been heavily skewed towards 'lower ability' students. Northwark Park became a specialist school and ability tests were introduced in order to secure a more 'balanced' intake. As a consequence, the school became over-subscribed in Year 7. However, it still had spare places in the other years, which meant that the school continued to be vulnerable to the selective and exclusionary practices of other schools in the local competitive arena.

Reviewing mixed ability

In 1992 the school conducted a review of its mixed-ability policy, which resulted in the science department introducing setting. All the other departments, apart from art and physical education, were to move to setting in subsequent years. Prior to the review, all classes were mixed-ability in all subjects and all years. The review can be understood as a response to the combination of a range of disciplinary mechanisms: open enrolment (i.e., parental choice), the publication of raw results in the form of league tables, the structure of national testing at Key Stages Three and Four,[13] the effects of under-resourcing on class sizes and special needs provision, the policy of Northwark LEA's inspectorate and the introduction of teacher appraisal:

13 The national curriculum identifies four 'key stages' of learning. At the end of each key stage children are assessed. The introduction of differential testing at Key Stages Three and Four means that teachers have to decide, some time in advance of the tests, at which level to enter their students. Key Stage Four refers to the period of a student's education between the ages of 14 and 16 and Key Stage Three to the 11 to 14 age group.

I think the ball game being as it is at the moment, where academic results are published in raw form, that we have to pay attention to that and try to improve our results. Now that may lead us to make decisions which we are not politically aligned to, but we are sort of, I'm talking about sort of mixed ability or do you go for streaming? Discussion is going on in the school at the moment, so to some extent some people would say that that is moving away from the comprehensive idea, others wouldn't . . . I think, to deliver the national curriculum in the best way, we may be forced into doing some kind of setting or grouping, especially higher up in the school because in Key Stage Four, we're being set differentiated papers.

(Acting deputy head)

Mixed ability is also on our agenda. We're reviewing it at the moment . . . not as a response to parents but because we don't think that we're doing it right at the moment. The national curriculum has made us review it really. I think it may well have an off shoot though, that it may make us attractive to parents . . . [The staff are] finding it more and more difficult, you see, resources have been cut, there's no doubt about it. With the national curriculum coming in there are more and more subjects which are say coping with that ability range within the classroom without the kind of support that you need is very difficult.

(Headteacher)

In other areas, as in science, they are now saying that they cannot possibly teach mixed-ability classes any more because they're having to cover completely different levels, so in a mixed ability class they'd have children at level six and other children who are at level two. So there is a move to go back to setting, which we've tried to resist.

(Head of special needs)

Whilst the introduction of setting in some subjects might have had the 'off shoot', as the headteacher put it, of attracting middle-class parents and might also have served to raise the academic performance of some children, there was clearly a downside with respect to the achievement of 'less able' children and children with special needs: 'you then get the development of the label of failure and the D-Stream culture. The movement that is there in the mixed-ability class is lost' (head of special needs).

This teacher's concerns about the association of setting with low teacher expectations of working-class and black children and restricted opportunities for these groups of students are supported by a significant body of research (e.g., Oakes 1990; Hallam and Toutounji 1996; Slavin 1996; Boaler 1997a; Sukhnandan and Lee 1998). As Sally Tomlinson has pointed out:

> Although ability is supposedly the major criterion for placement in subject and examination levels, ability is an ambiguous concept and school conceptions of ability can be affected by perceptions that pupils are members of particular social or ethnic groups and by the behaviour of individual pupils. Factors related to class, gender, ethnicity, and behaviour *can* be shown to affect the placement of pupils at option time, even those of similar ability.
>
> (Tomlinson 1987: 106)

The integration of children with special needs

Like many state schools since the publication of the Warnock Report (DES 1978), Northwark Park had progressively moved away from the remedial approach to special needs provision, where children with special needs were mainly withdrawn from mainstream classes and taught a virtually separate curriculum, towards a more integrated approach with an emphasis on in-class support. But there were signs in Northwark Park that the trend towards integration had begun to recede because of market forces and the associated shift of resources away from children with special needs.

I have already pointed to the introduction of setting in some subjects, which constitutes an obvious barrier to integration. I have also referred to the contraction of the special needs department resulting in a reduced capacity for in-class support for children with special needs. In addition to these developments, the reorganisation of special needs provision in the local authority as a whole, whilst presented by the authority as a policy designed to enhance integration, in practice meant that off-site support was also reduced. This gave rise to fears that: 'there probably won't even be enough to cover the statutory work that we do . . . No doubt there will be children next year who have got statements who won't have the support they are legally entitled to' (head of special needs). Such concerns are by no means peculiar to Northwark Park (Gewirtz *et al.* 1995).

But it was not just a shortage of resources and a local authority apparently more concerned about challenging the 'able' than stretching the 'less able' that put pressure on the ability of the school to provide for special needs adequately. There were other disciplinary mechanisms at work here, which functioned to stunt the development of integrative policies. The desire that the school should be attractive to 'motivated' parents with 'able' children combined with inadequate resourcing to operate as a disincentive for good special needs provision and the integration of children with special needs. The deputy head commented:

> It's a fairly contentious thing to say but I think special educational needs could suffer. I think people will be less tolerant, because that sort of provision is expensive, so it's eating up your money and your time, and if you're being asked to produce a good set of examination results, then you want as much of your resourcing as possible to be directed at that.

And the head of special needs gave a very specific example of where consideration of image and resourcing became significant influences in the school's thinking about the admission of two children with severe learning difficulties:

> Actually this school has got a good reputation for special needs. Primary schools, when they come to advise parents of children with difficulties will say, 'well Northwark Park is good, they seem to look after the kids who've got special needs very well' . . . Next year, for instance, we're having a kid who's got Down's Syndrome. He's going to be joining us and then there was . . . another one with another, not Down's but something else, who also thought, ah yes, Northwark Park and we thought, well no, we can't take two. This is going to be enough having one child with that level of need and integrating – I mean it's such a new thing for us, we can't deal with two, we just can't handle it, we're going to be stretched enough as it is. But luckily the parents have decided to go elsewhere . . . But we were beginning to think, oh my gosh, are we going to start getting a reputation, 'ah yes, Northwark Park, they integrate students with these difficulties'. And then, you know, what effect does that have on the perception of parents with that school, when they come to want a school for their band one kid, do they send them to that school?

So in the area of special needs, educational considerations were beginning to be subordinated to commercial ones. Once again then, funding shortages, local authority policy towards provision for the 'less able', *per capita* funding, national testing, the publication of league tables of raw scores and the subsequent concern to attract more 'able' children into the school combined to form a disciplinary framework which worked against the culture of comprehensivism and, in this particular instance, integration.

The question of exclusions

Governors and staff at Northwark Park had observed an increase in the rate of permanent exclusions from other local schools:

> That's what's differentiating between the schools that are assertive and feel that they are oversubscribed. [They] have no hesitation in chucking kids out on very tenuous evidence, you know, to encourage the rest of the school community.
>
> (Chair of governors)

> The exclusion rate has gone up considerably. You know, to expel a student was quite a rare thing. It's now become commonplace, and in fairly large numbers. And then when they're excluded, they just sort of hike round the authority from one school to another. We've just excluded a boy who has already been excluded from two other schools . . . [T]he pressures on schools to produce the goods in terms of academic success has made them less willing to spend their resources and their time and their energy on students who almost dissipate their energies, on students who are just trying to mess the system up.
>
> (Deputy head)

Local and national statistics would appear to support these impressions, with permanent exclusions rising and a disproportionate number of black boys being excluded (Gillborn and Gipps 1996). Whilst local oversubscribed schools were able to exclude, Northwark Park was under pressure to accept the excluded:[14]

> Our school is attracting a very large number of usually expelled, displaced fifteen year olds, who've missed the option level, so

---

14 This continued to be the case even after the introduction of selection in 1998. Because the school was not full to capacity in every year, it was required to accept students excluded from other local schools. This was not a requirement that applied to the local foundation (formerly grant-maintained) schools.

they're coming into our school. Our exam results as a result will be quite seriously affected by the number who've joined us after the beginning of Year 10 and therefore are almost bound to have a restricted exam potential.

(Chair of governors)

There were divergent views within the school about the educational merits and demerits of permanent exclusion. The Education Welfare Officer (EWO) was opposed to exclusion on the grounds that it does not benefit the excluded child because the source of the problem which leads to exclusion in the first place is not confronted: 'if a child is not attending because they don't have, you know, meaningful relationships with children in the school, or they don't know the staff very well . . . moving them to another school is not going to solve that'.

There was a group of teachers within the school, however, who wanted the school's exclusion policy to be tightened up. At an in-service training day, in which the school development plan was discussed, some members of staff were critical of senior management for not taking up effectively complaints about a core of disruptive students who were seen to be absorbing a disproportionate amount of teacher time and consequently damaging the learning of other children. At the feedback session on the day, there was a heated discussion between the head and a number of teachers about this group of students, which focused on the issue of exclusions:

One teacher pointed out that these children were disrupting other students on a regular basis and another commented that the number of GCSE grade As in one particular class was lowered because of the presence of a disruptive pupil in that class. The head reported that she had presented to the governors the exclusion figures since January and that they thought they were high. A teacher responded: 'They don't have to deal with them. Let them come into the classes and deal with it'.

(Observation notes)

There was clearly a resource dimension to the arguments of these teachers. If class sizes had been smaller and there had been less pressure on teacher and senior management time and resources more generally, then other strategies might have been more easily found to deal with this group of children. But on the whole, as far as the teaching staff were concerned, the debate was essentially about the *educational,* or at least classroom management, advantages or disadvantages of exclusion.

At management level, however, it would seem that on the issue of exclusion, as in other areas, educational questions were being increasingly subordinated to commercial, market-oriented ones. The debate within management about whether or not to exclude was centred on the question of whether it was a good or bad marketing strategy and about the financial implications of excluding. Oversubscribed schools can easily replace their excluded students with students on their waiting lists. But if Northwark Park excluded, they were unlikely to get a replacement and would lose the money attached to the excluded pupil: 'I mean each child now is worth money and you've got to be pretty desperate to actually suggest a parent changes school for a child' (head of Year 7).

Belonging to a local system

It was argued at Northwark Park that an essential part of being a comprehensive school was belonging to a local system of comprehensive schools. Yet the local system in Northwark was dissolving. The break up of the ILEA was perhaps the first nail in the coffin but the market and the grant-maintained schools policy accelerated the dissolution. Many Northwark teachers were trying to resist the fragmentation that the market fosters. The head of the sixth form at Northwark Park was part of a group of Northwark heads of sixth form trying to maintain links:

> I don't like being in a situation where we're competing for students. Luckily my colleagues in sixth forms in other schools, locally, we've more or less agreed that we won't poach from each other's schools so that if a fifth year student from another school applies to the sixth form here, I would get back to his or her school, and tell them that is the case. As I say, we've got a general agreement, there is a small group of us . . . but there's one school in particular in the LEA that seems to take anybody, and has always been the first one to try and poach. That's their policy. It's a bigger school and some people think the best school, but that's been going on for some while.

But however much individual teachers would have liked to continue cooperating with other schools, the odds were increasingly against it happening because the new deregulated structure of school provision is not conducive to cooperation. This is mainly because it encourages competition, which has led to the souring of relations between some schools:

> Another school which prides itself in the sheer number of band ones it manages to get in, and it does it absolutely immorally . . . and . . . it's full up, it's oversubscribed, it is an oversubscribed school. And they used to take their full quotas of band ones, twos and threes, as they used to be called . . . but if a child leaves, and they have a space available . . . now you can offer that space to anybody and they actually ring round, and I have had children poached from [the school] – 'Oh we now have a space available . . . are you still interested . . . ?' And they're totally immoral and I hope they suffer in hell for it later . . . because I think they damage more children than they've done service by.
>
> (Teacher governor)

Also, once schools opted out, professional contact between teachers in different sectors became difficult to maintain:

> We have official meetings at the Teachers' Centre about four or five times a year and then unofficial contacts . . . But the group is narrowing because of the opting out.
>
> (Head of sixth form)

> When I came with the previous head we were both, we were members of SHA [Secondary Heads Association] and we would meet with other schools regularly, again all the schools from Northwark would be represented, because we're all more or less [SHA] members and they would discuss mutual problems and things. These meetings more or less no longer exist, and if they do they're poorly attended, and I don't think there is any rift between heads as such, but there is not the unity that there was. Maybe there's a feeling of mutual suspicion.
>
> (Deputy head)[15]

And, of course, the fragmentation of the local system of schooling has very obvious effects on the pupils, as is apparent in the following example given by the head of sixth form:

> I don't agree with formula funding. I think it's not the way to fund education for a start. It's a very stark choice. You know, one

student is worth so many pounds, there's a very strong pressure, therefore, to accept students who would be better advised to go elsewhere. And sometimes we have truthfully, we have had one or two in the sixth form who perhaps should not have been in the sixth form, but they were here because they wanted to be and it was very useful to have them to boost the numbers, and boost our income. We still don't do it as much as some institutions I won't name, but there are local places that will take anybody. It's not quite as easy as that, there are enumeration days during the year so it's not quite who you've got on roll for the first day of the year and after that you can say goodbye, and get the money, but nevertheless there is an element of creative accounting, if you like.

(Head of sixth form)

Conclusion

The case of Northwark Park illustrates how certain values, interests and needs are privileged in the education market place and how others are marginalised via the systematic restructuring of school provision. The market is not a neutral mechanism of resource allocation, nor is it apolitical: it is a form of 'ordered competition' (Hayek 1980) with *particular* social and economic goals embedded in it. We have seen that the market functions as a disciplinary mechanism via the provision of incentives and disincentives. Open enrolment and *per capita* funding, poor resourcing, the testing of children at four key stages and the publication of league tables of those results are crucial components of that mechanism. Research on parental choice indicates that exam results are only one of several criteria seen by parents as being important in helping them decide on a secondary school for their children (David *et al.* 1994; Gewirtz *et al.* 1995; Woods *et al.* 1998). Yet the publication of league tables of results and the publicity

15 It is yet to be seen whether the re-incorporation of grant-maintained schools into the LEA will facilitate the re-emergence of collaborative relations between schools, or whether the continued existence of the market and competition will make the rifts that have been created too difficult to repair. However, by 1999, although New Labour's Excellence in Cities programme had, according to Northwark Park's chair of governors, forced schools to talk to each other, relations between schools remained competitive. (Excellence in Cities is an initiative that channels additional funds into urban schools to be spent on specific projects, for example, programmes for 'gifted and talented' students and learning mentors for 'disaffected' young people.)

surrounding their publication mean that schools are paying particular attention to test results. Low levels of funding mean that schools are pressured into maximising their results in the cheapest ways possible. Admitting only those students who are likely to perform well in tests and excluding those who are likely to perform badly are the most cost-effective means for (oversubscribed) schools to boost their positions in the league tables; and setting is a cheaper way of organising learning than mixed-ability grouping. Another element of the disciplinary mechanism, which has further encouraged the more widespread adoption of setting practices, has been the introduction of differential testing at Key Stages Three and Four (see footnote 13).

Northwark Park is a 'critical case' that illustrates how difficult it is for schools to resist the discipline imposed by the market. It is a school whose staff and governors were ideologically committed to comprehensive education. Thus, if there were any potential for strategies to be developed that would enable schools to retain immunity from market pressures, one would have expected Northwark Park to have developed and utilised them. But, as we have seen, in order to survive in the market place, the school was having to consider cultivating a more middle-class intake. And by 1998, the school had abandoned two of the key components of its comprehensivism – namely, mixed-ability teaching and being non-selective.

The case of Northwark Park also illustrates how the market rewards positioning rather than principles and encourages commercial rather than educational decision-making. This is evidenced, in particular, by the staff's comments on exclusions, integration and sixth-form provision. This reflects a fundamental value shift in the English education system (Gewirtz *et al.* 1995). Within the post-welfarist policy environment, concern for social justice is being replaced by concern for institutional survival, collectivism with individualism, cooperation with suspicion and need with expediency. However, it is important to reiterate that this shift is not smooth and nor has it gone uncontested. Those involved in schools are differently located along the 'values spectrum', which ranges from 'comprehensivism' on one end to 'marketism' on the other (Gewirtz *et al.* 1995): whilst some governors and teachers are relatively accepting of the drift towards setting and selection, viewing these developments as necessary evils, others are more stubbornly resistant to the retreat from comprehensivist practices and values that these developments are seen to represent.

4 Stress in the staffroom

The reconstruction of teachers' work

Chapters 2 and 3 have explored the consequences of post-welfarist policies for the management of schools and some of the ethical dilemmas prompted by the marketisation of schooling. I now want to delve a little deeper into the life of schools by examining how teachers are experiencing the shifts in management practices and values that have been considered in these earlier chapters.

Teachers' work has always been constrained or controlled – for example, by the timetable, student groupings, the allocation of space, examination syllabuses, textbook availability and authoritarian headteachers. But increased competitiveness, target setting and performance monitoring, and the narrowing of definitions of performance associated with the new managerialism can be seen to represent aspects of a qualitatively different regime of constraint and control in schools. In particular, as we saw in Chapter 2, the competitive environment and the budget- and performance-oriented climate of schooling encourages the borrowing of 'macho' styles of management from the private sector. Within this new regime, neo-Taylorist management practices coexist with post-Taylorist ones. Thus, there is a clear separation between policy formulation and execution: a diminution of teacher control (and indeed headteacher control) over decisions about the ultimate goals and objectives of their work, and pressure on teachers to become increasingly preoccupied with the technical aspects of meeting aims and targets set elsewhere. There is a shift, in other words from a *substantive* to *technical* rationality in schools (Considine 1988; Bottery 1992) (see Chapter 2). At the same time, there is a post-Taylorist emphasis on 'flexibility' (Lawn 1996), 'teamwork' and, in some cases, moves towards flatter management structures. These are general trends. There are, however, very clear differences to be found in the management regimes of different schools. A strong market position, for example, can provide the latitude for a more democratic management style (see Chapter 5).

So, what effect is all of this having on the work that teachers do? A 1991 International Labour Office (ILO) report on teachers' work in over forty countries noted that:

> The main trends in hours worked over the past decade are defined by a number of common features. First, though the number of actual teaching hours in contact with students has remained static, or even decreased slightly in most countries . . . the overall workload of teachers appears to have increased. The main growth areas of work are administrative duties to conform to additional rules and regulations, and the attention devoted to unruly pupils. Secondly, work in the evenings and on weekends remains a steady, though irregular, component of teachers' working time . . . Thirdly, stress and time pressures increasingly characterise the working day of most teachers.
>
> (ILO 1991: 84–86)

A number of surveys carried out in Britain (e.g. NAS/UWT 1990 and 1991; Lowe 1991; Campbell and St J. Neill 1994a; STRB 2000a and 2000b) suggest that developments here mirror the international trends reported by the ILO – an increase in the overall number of hours that teachers work and a broadening of tasks that teachers are expected to carry out, with an increased emphasis on administration.

Such quantification of the changing nature of teachers' work is useful but is limited in a number of ways and needs to be complemented by a more theoretically-informed qualitative analysis. Survey data gives us little idea of the implications of these changes for pedagogical practice and the social relations of schooling. Nor do we get any picture of the emotional consequences of these changes – what they *feel* like for teachers and how they are experienced *differently* by teachers in different schools, different departments and different status locations. Also, *measures* of change can be relatively meaningless without a more detailed picture of what is involved. For example, Campbell and St J. Neill's (1994a) data indicate that teachers were interacting with each other more in the early 1990s than they were 15 years earlier but in itself this finding tells us very little. What we need to know, and what the quantitative research cannot tell us, is how the *nature* of these interactions is changing. This chapter examines the changing nature of intensification associated with the marketisation and managerialisation of school provision, drawing on interviews carried out with teachers in four secondary schools.[16]

The changing nature of intensification

> There are days when I leave here and I haven't stood still for a second and I haven't had one minute to myself to even go to the toilet or to just think.
>
> (Jackie Green, English teacher, Ruskin School)

The survey research cited above indicates an accelerated intensification towards the end of the twentieth century. Teachers worked on average approximately seven more hours a week in the early 1990s than they had worked in the early 1970s (Campbell and St J. Neill 1994a) and the length of the working week for teachers continued to rise throughout the 1990s (STRB 2000a). However, it is important to recognise that the labour process of teaching has always been intense. Thus, there is little doubt that most teachers working in the *welfarist* era would be able to empathise with Jackie Green, cited above. What appears to be different in the *post-welfarist* era is the pattern and texture of intensification; that is, the *nature* of the tasks that are absorbing increased quantities of teacher time and emotional labour, and the climate of surveillance within which those tasks have to be carried out. The growing emphasis on formalised assessment, target-setting and performance monitoring is generating huge amounts of paperwork. In addition, particular subject areas are having to make regular and repeated changes to their syllabuses in response to changing external requirements. There is also a perception in schools of increased behavioural difficulties amongst the student population (perhaps relating to the wider socio-economic and policy shifts associated with

16 The interviews were conducted as part of the ESRC-funded study, 'Schools, Cultures and Values' (see Footnote 3). The schools were all located in different London authorities. Beatrice Webb is an undersubscribed, inner-London, almost exclusively working-class, co-educational comprehensive school (see Chapters 2 and 5 for more details). Ruskin is a popular inner-London co-educational, comprehensive school not far from Beatrice Webb but more mixed in terms of the social class of its intake (see Chapter 5 for more details). Fletcher is an oversubscribed outer-London co-educational, socially mixed comprehensive worried about its disproportionate intake of 'lower ability' students. Martineau is a very popular outer-London socially mixed, girls' school, which became grant-maintained and selective over the course of our research. Pseudonyms are used throughout. See Appendix for details of the research methods used.

post-welfarism) so that, in line with the ILO findings, many teachers reported to us that increased quantities of their time were taken up with dealing with 'difficult' students. These stresses and strains are compounded in oversubscribed schools by overcrowding and in undersubscribed ones by a shortage of resources manifested in poor physical conditions, insufficient learning and language support, and a shortage of textbooks and other equipment deemed essential. An increasingly competitive climate both across and within schools, and heightened forms of surveillance, mean that teachers feel under growing pressure to perform and conform. All of these things appear to be having a number of important consequences. I discuss these under three headings: emotional consequences; consequences for social relations; and pedagogical consequences. The separation is in reality somewhat artificial – all three kinds of consequences are, of course, overlapping and inter-related.

Emotional consequences

The more direct forms of control, which are integral to the new managerial regimes operating within post-welfarist schools, place enormous strains on teachers, which were vividly conveyed to us in the interviews. Teachers referred, for example, to the 'manic grind' and 'frenetic pace' of work and to being 'squeezed dry'. How surveillance regimes operate and the climate of frenzied activity and fear they can generate are captured in the following comments by Karen Sargent, a head of cluster at Martineau School:

K. Sargent: If you've got a bottom set, you're never going to get very good work out of them, you've got to sort of keep it coming, and I think that feeling that we're all accountable, and we're all expected to teach to the best of our ability – Obviously the core subjects have got the SATs as the real – I don't know what you'd call it – something hanging over their heads, which they know, if their class dips . . . that would be terrible.

Interviewer: How would that be realised?

K. Sargent: I think actually the heads of those three clusters would look at the results, class-by-class, and they would see if any class was below expectations and that teacher would have to answer for it. We are all very accountable then for our exam results. So obviously you start with Year 7, trying to get them on the right lines, knowing that in five years time they'll be doing GCSE, the results will be published, they will be expected to be either at or above the national average, or very close to, and if they're severely below, then you would expect to be called to account, and nobody likes that. So that affects our practice. And even if you know you've got a pretty poor quality group, you want to be able to demonstrate . . . the classroom teachers here would want to demonstrate to their heads of subject, to me, to our senior team link, and if necessary to Mrs Carnegie [the headteacher] herself, the fact that we'd done absolutely everything, run revision sessions (but we couldn't make them turn up) we'd given them all these revision guides (but we can't make them read them) you know, we'd done absolutely everything we can. And then if you'd come here [at the] beginning of the Easter term, there's this . . . frenzy at lunchtime with geography revision and history revision and sociology revision. We're all . . . pushing them forward to try and get them through.

(Head of cluster, Martineau School)

There are three important points to note about this quote. First, it represents a lucid description of one aspect of how *performativity* works in education and more specifically of how the values embedded within the PWEPC become internalised within schools. As Stephen Ball has noted, performativity in education functions 'as a disciplinary system of judgements, classifications and targets towards which schools and teachers must strive and against and through which they are evaluated' (Ball 1998). Like the other headteachers in the study, one of Mrs Carnegie's (Head of Martineau) responses to league tables, inspection and the generally competitive climate within which most schools are now operating was to install hierarchically structured internal systems of accountability. In the case of Martineau School, classroom teachers are accountable to 'heads of cluster', who in turn are accountable to the 'senior teacher link' and the headteacher. These clear lines of accountability, coupled with appraisal systems, effectively regulate the work of teachers, ensuring that the values of the performance-driven market are institutionalised to the extent that they penetrate classroom practice.

The second important point to note about Karen Sargent's comments is her construction of low-attaining groups of students as 'poor quality'. Clearly this is not a simple case of market values and, more specifically, the commodification of children, permeating the classroom. Such 'academicist' constructions certainly pre-date the market, having long been a feature of hegemonic teacher discourses. However, by placing such a great emphasis on exam performance, post-welfarist educational regimes certainly appear to reinforce the differential valuing of students according to their levels of academic attainment, an issue I will return to below.

Finally, Karen Sargent's comments capture the stressful nature of constantly having to ensure and demonstrate satisfactory levels of student performance. However, it is not just the workload and the surveillance that is stressful. The nature of the tasks that are now occupying teachers and the perceived loss of control involved also have emotional consequences. For example, a number of the teachers interviewed expressed resentment at having to spend so much of their time recording and monitoring students' work in the formal way now required of them. Such work is viewed as a distraction from what they see as the *real* work of teaching – i.e., preparing lessons, interacting with students both within and outside the classroom, and marking. For many teachers an integral part of their 'real' work involves focusing their energies on children across the ability range but, as I discuss below, teachers are increasingly being encouraged to target particular groups of students. The teachers we interviewed also expressed resentment at having to expend energy working to objectives, targets and requirements set elsewhere, particularly where those objectives conflicted with their own. Jackie Green, again:

> I'm beginning to feel much more impotent then I ever have really. There's much less control over . . . the texts that I choose and the methods I want to use.
>
> (English teacher, Ruskin School)

And Janice Lee, a head of year at Fletcher School:

> Good teaching is about teachers being given some autonomy, some opportunity to experiment, to try new things out and there's not very much of that anymore . . . I get very cross when somebody publishes a pamphlet saying, you will make sure you've got this, that and the other . . . It's become too prescriptive . . . you've got to make sure that this, this, this, and this is done and tick this box and fill in this form. It's just like, what am I doing . . . do they need me or a robot?

In order to protect their students and what they consider to be their *real* work from work which is imposed upon them, teachers have to expend enormous quantities of energy:

> I think it's a case of, either you accept you work seven days a week or else your teaching goes down . . . I still try and find the energy to keep my teaching exciting, but it's hard, very hard.
>
> (Janice Lee, Fletcher School)

This kind of approach to work is indeed a product of teacher-conscientiousness (Campbell and St J. Neill 1994a; Hargreaves 1994) but, as Julian Smith, an English teacher at Ruskin School, pointed out, it is also a product of new forms of control. In responding, conscientiously, to the structured demands of the PWEPC, teachers can become the repositories of accumulated stress:

> How does it effect the children? I think we try to make sure it doesn't but . . . in the same way that toxins in water accumulate up the food chains, the thing at the top gets the most toxin because it is eating lots of little things that accumulate in it. Because we decide that we are not gonna . . . actually pass on the stress to students it then accumulates in us. So the government passes it to SCAA,[17] SCAA pass it to the heads of schools, heads of schools pass it to us and we are not going to pass it on so the stress stops and piles up on us.

Consequences for social relations

The PWEPC appears to be having consequences for social relations throughout school life. As noted in Chapter 2, there continues to be a gap in perspective between senior staff with a greater concern with the kinds of activities associated with running a business – like balancing the budget, recruitment and marketing – and teaching staff with a greater concern with classroom-based practices – like curriculum coverage, classroom control, student needs and record keeping. The increase in more direct forms of surveillance has obvious effects on relationships between management and staff (Reay 1998). There are also consequences for horizontal relations amongst staff. Whilst it

---

17 Schools Curriculum and Assessment Authority (SCAA) – a quango set up to regulate the national curriculum and its assessment. It has since been renamed as the Qualifications and Curriculum Authority.

seemed to be the case in the schools researched that teachers were meeting more often, and many teachers complained of being overburdened with meetings, there was at the same time a perception of a *decline in the sociability of school life*. The meetings that were taking up increasing quantities of teacher time were working in large part to agendas set by senior managers who were in turn, to a significant degree, working to agendas set by the requirements of the PWEPC. Individual subject areas found themselves short of time to discuss the *real* work of the department and there was less opportunity for inter-departmental collaboration over curriculum issues, where previously that kind of collaboration had occurred. There also appeared to be less opportunity for informal socialising amongst staff:

> One is struggling on one's own . . . battling against all the paperwork.
>
> (Art teacher, Fletcher School)

> My own best work was produced in collaboration with other areas like drama, dance and music, and they weren't timetabled, we just found our own time. We were inspired to teach in that way.
>
> (Head of art, Ruskin School)

> If you go to our staffroom at lunchtime you won't find anyone in it, nobody at all . . . Jesus, years ago, that was the main collective point. Now what happens is that everybody . . . stays in their own [department], working.
>
> (Head of year, Beatrice Webb School)

The decline in sociability was, in part, a product of time shortage but it was also related to the growing inter-departmental competitiveness of school life. Conflict between departments, what Hargreaves (1994) calls Balkanisation, is a product of competitive bidding for resources and competition for exam results, and to varying degrees it is intentionally fostered by headteacher strategies of divide and rule (Reay 1998).

It was the perception of a number of teachers that relationships between teachers and students were also in the process of being reworked. A combination of larger class sizes, the expansion of paperwork and the growing emphasis on performance as opposed to process meant that increasingly there was a pressure for intimate and complicated relationships to dissolve and become more distant and formal:

J. Cooper:	The ability to work with children on a more individual basis is going slightly as well. I mean you used to see a lot of staff working with children in the lunchtimes, not on an organised basis but on a . . . sort of, 'Come in and I'll help you with this, that and the other'. That used to happen a lot, it doesn't happen so much any more.
Interviewer:	What do you think is lost from not having so much informal contact?
J. Cooper:	I think . . . the sort of relationship between the teacher and the child . . . the sort of trust relationship that you can build up between them, because it's actually very difficult in a class to build up a good relationship with the kids, particularly when . . . the classes are large . . . I personally have found that I'm not as close to the children as I used to be.

(Julie Cooper, head of faculty, Fletcher School)

Pedagogical consequences

In describing the emotional consequences of post-welfarism for teachers' work, I referred to the stresses involved in protecting the *real* work of teaching. However, not all teachers do feel able to protect what they see as their real work as vigorously as they would like. This is especially the case in schools where resources are scarce and where many of the students are in need of high levels of learning support. A number of teachers working in such circumstances perceive a general decline in the vitality and creativity of their teaching:

> I'm going to kill myself, I'm going to be dead by Christmas if I'm trying to do great . . . big outreaching things which I used to. I used to be able to set up debates and give them half an hour or so . . . to have counterpoint and all that sort of thing. I'm not able to do that now so I don't think my teaching is quite so imaginative.
>
> (Head of department, Beatrice Webb School)

There were teachers in all four schools who reported *a narrowing of focus in their work*. This narrowing was manifested in a number of ways, which will be discussed below: pressure on extra-curricula activity, increased emphasis on exams and outcomes, an increased focus on targeting pupils and the differential fortunes of school subjects. These forms of narrowing were reflected in, and reproduced by, the return to more traditional sorting mechanisms within schools, i.e., setting. First, although the headteachers were attempting to convey the impression to parents of expanded extra-curricular provision, there appeared to be a decline in what might be termed *organic* extra-curricular activity, by which I mean activities initiated by teachers rather than imposed upon them:

> I'm squeezed dry for the working week. I've got these reports to write and these assessments to look through. The paperwork that's been generated by . . . the DFE [Department for Education] in terms of monitoring . . . achievement, it takes up so much time that people rightly think, 'Well, I've done my whack . . . It's interfering with my personal life and time outside the school so hugely that I don't really feel . . . inclined to do . . . extra things for the students after school'.
>
> (George O'Brien, head of year, Ruskin School)

There were also accounts of a more utilitarian, exam-oriented approach to teaching, with less emphasis on responding to the interests of the children, the cultivation of relationships and the *process* of learning, and more emphasis on learning *outcomes*:

> I've had to become a lot more aware of students working under timed conditions . . . to see what they can do in an exam . . . That is increasingly eating away at what I would call effective teaching and learning . . . it's more of a mental preparation for timed work than it is about learning . . . There's less flexibility [to pursue issues the students show an interest in] . . . I'm much more conscious of the clock ticking and therefore I am very, very reluctant to have anything interrupt that time plan.
>
> (Jackie Green, English teacher, Ruskin School)

> You are looking over your shoulder at the other schools' results and there is . . . a definite rivalry there, and we know that they are raw scores and really quite unreliable if you balance them with . . . social class intake and all the other elements that . . . give a realistic picture of the school, but . . . there is that pressure you feel, that's not being stated openly but it's kind of unwritten, that you must keep those scores up as high as possible. And that involves . . . more utilitarian planning and teaching . . . and that's what your main goal is with the kids to the exclusion of all else really.
>
> (George O'Brien, head of year, Ruskin School)

I think we have become more of an exams factory, and . . . you think much more about what kind of objectives you're meeting . . . In some ways it's tightened us up but I think . . . we've lost a bit of flair . . . I think I've lost . . . the chance you have . . . of taking a tangent . . . when you want to . . . the chance to . . . feel, . . . I can actually follow this through a bit more – you know, or, sod that part of the course, I'll follow this through . . . which we some-times . . . did, . . . but now . . . our schemes of work are pretty much laid out week by week . . . and we try and hammer through them . . . I used to have more time to . . . devise . . . what I would call 'creative lessons' . . . When I was at [my last school] . . . there was a real pressure on you to come up with really good lessons . . . but that was the pressure, to come up with really good lessons . . . The good lesson was so you had a good lesson, it wasn't so that you had a good exam result or anything like that.

(Andrew Martin, head of year, Ruskin School)

Dan Rose, head of art at Ruskin, vividly captured a perceived shift from a vibrant expressive, relationship-centred culture of teaching to a narrow instrumentalist, utilitarian one:

[The 1960s] was a very sort of exciting period and the students were producing very gutsy exciting work, which was not so much exam orientated and was not so much art school, miniature art school orientated type of work produced. So I felt that it was a very mean-ingful period, and through art we could reach out, create relation-ships, and also create the atmosphere where we could see students grow within our relationships with them. . . . [It's a] little bit more artificial now, it's all judged on paperwork and how well students perform in examinations – and I'm part of the system I'm afraid, I haven't stepped out of it . . . But I reflect on that period as a very happy, a very exciting period.

Dan Rose connected these changes, and his own reluctant accommo-dation to the 'new times' in education, to heightened and more direct forms of surveillance within the school imposed by external demands:

It's been a gradual change really. I suppose in the national curricu-lum, or just before that when people began to – well, to put it bluntly, people began to look in one's cabinets and drawers to see what classes have produced, to try and analyse what is going on. I think one then had to concentrate on a different form of teaching – how much have they produced, assessment and . . . all that. So one had to begin to teach in a different way, to show artefacts, to show results.

Linked to this emphasis on outcomes is a pressure to focus on the needs of *particular groups of students*. In all the case-study schools there is now a targeting of so-called borderline students – those at the threshold of attaining C grades at GCSE:

> The idea is you pull anyone you think is gonna be a D up to a C, there's pressure for that, that's where the pressure lies . . . the expectation is that I will be giving revision classes, particularly targeted at those who are at D level, or E and D level, to get Cs, which I think is fair enough, but it is a pressure . . . It's my first exam group. I am conscious of them doing well. If they do badly [that will] reflect on me . . . rather than the . . . calibre of the girls in the group . . . I think really, yes, I'm raising the standards of a few, purely for the exam grade percentages, not the whole group.
> (Geoff Wright, maingrade teacher, Martineau School)

Just in this short quote, Geoff Wright used the word 'pressure' three times. It is a term that arose frequently in teachers' accounts of their work.

At Beatrice Webb School, where in 1996 only 9 per cent of students got five or more A–Cs at GCSE and where almost two-thirds of the students are categorised as bilingual, Matthew Peters, a science teacher, described a situation in which he felt pressurised to focus on the one or two children in his class who may have got a C or above at GCSE: 'At the end of the day', he said, 'I've got to get somebody to get a C and above, because that's what's counted on the school's percentage and league tables'. This forced him to adopt didactic teaching methods with very little practical work. Such methods were wholly inappropriate for the majority of the students in the class, some of whom were unable to read and write in any language. The inadequacy of resources in the school – which was linked to low subscription rates and a funding formula that takes little account of student need – meant that the school could not afford to provide its students with the levels of classroom support they needed. Given this situation, it is very difficult to see how, for most of the students, any significant educational benefit could be gained from their presence in the classroom.

Dan Rose was similarly candid about the consequences of a focus on outcomes and attainment in the context of diminishing resources.

Whilst those students he described as talented might have benefited from what he referred to as 'a Thatcherite preoccupation with results and excellence', the new regime of performativity appeared to have left him weary and without the emotional strength to channel the compassion he once had into the students who, he felt, most needed his help:

> One hasn't got the time to deal with the ones who – the students who hadn't had the background, who hadn't had books at home, who'd never been to an exhibition. If you want to cater for that I think one needs [a] different emphasis and [a] different approach entirely. You need several people in the room, just one teacher can't really manage. You have to teach collectively in a way . . . And hence they fall by the wayside, in my opinion. I mean you try your best – the job is exhausting, and in the end you only want to help, psychologically you only want to help the students who are interested and want to do the work. You don't want to delve into the difficult area of trying to do a one to one with that sort of student . . . That is the real truth of it, and that's unfortunate and I feel that . . . my teaching did involve that sort of compassion to help the students who needed that particular help.
>
> (Head of art, Ruskin School)

For many teachers (possibly *particularly*, although clearly not exclusively, in urban settings) work satisfaction and enjoyment is derived from interacting with varied sets of students. Within these interactions a whole range of types of achievement are valued. But increasingly many of the teachers we interviewed felt under pressure to focus on particular groups of students and to adopt narrow, academic conceptions of performance.

There are also specific pedagogical consequences of expanding school intakes. Overcrowding alters the social space of the classroom, encouraging the use of more traditional pedagogical approaches. For English and humanities teachers, who tend towards more active, responsive and discussion-oriented pedagogies, the impact of larger class sizes is felt most acutely and within these classrooms we appear to be seeing a return to more didactic and static pedagogical practices – as one teacher put it, 'you have to do a lot more talk and chalk':

> Sometimes you've got 29 Year 11s in a room that's barely [the size of] two of these [by these he meant the 'learning support' room

where we were doing the interview, which was a small box room about eight foot square]. And they hate it and it's smelly and hot, and . . . [there's] very little manoeuvre in terms of desk formation so you've got a very static kind of teaching style.

(Learning support teacher, Ruskin School)

My Year 10 class is 32 kids, I teach in a tiny room, if we're using maps and things I have to have kids working in the corridor. And I don't think I'm as adventurous as I'd like to be. If I had a bigger room or I had less kids I'd be able to do more.

(Andrew Martin, head of year, Ruskin School)

Difficulties are compounded in English and humanities by the imposition of an Anglo-centric curriculum, a statutory reduction in the proportion of coursework allowed and a return to more assessment by examination:

We've gone from 50 per cent exam . . . 50 per cent coursework A level – we're not allowed to do that anymore because of the government's demands, so this year it's 80 per cent exam, 20 per cent coursework. It means that I have to do a lot more spoonfeeding because . . . you have to prepare certain sorts of structures and formulae that kids can approach literature questions on an exam paper with, whereas with the coursework element you could be a lot more exploratory, a lot more adventurous in the kind of text you chose . . . and it's narrowed their literary experience.

(George O'Brien, head of year, Ruskin School)

Now because of the national curriculum, we're teaching issues which aren't necessarily dry but they're all in the same area, they're all on Britain and British history, with one or two exceptions, whereas in the past we would be able to look at issues which I think would engage the students much more, and you could actually not just be teaching them in a sort of stereotyped way, white middle-class British history . . . You'd actually be able to engage the students we have, and yet we can't do that any more, so I think it's becoming harder and harder, and I guess as a school we need to look at ways of somehow negating the national curriculum in that sense and actually being able to . . . engage the students . . . so for example I'm producing a new Year 9 course which is – we're going to call Humanities but it's going to be basically political, social and moral issues, and what we intend to do there is try and build up the curriculum for Year 9. We're actually looking at issues which we think will engage the students and actually do some of the things which we haven't been able to do because of the national curriculum.

(John Edwards, head of faculty, Ruskin School)

The relatively healthy budget at oversubscribed Ruskin enables John Edwards to preserve his *real* work by creating an alternative curriculum in this way. Those trying to do similar things at Beatrice Webb, with its poor resourcing and inadequate learning support, face a greater uphill struggle. In any case, for most teachers at Beatrice Webb, the concerns were far more immediate than developing alternatives to the national curriculum. The over-riding preoccupations of the majority of those interviewed were with problems of student behaviour, the management of the school and simply getting by on a shoestring budget.[18]

Another way in which the narrowing of focus is evidenced is in the shifting fortunes of non-core curriculum subjects. For example, drama tends to be regarded as an image-boosting subject, popular amongst middle-class clientele and, therefore, worthy of investment. Sociology, on the other hand, is not seen as particularly appealing to significant numbers of middle-class parents of students of compulsory school-age and is, thus, seen to be dispensable in the utilitarian, competitive era of post-welfarism.

The PWEPC has also contributed to a return to more traditional sorting mechanisms within schools. Setting is not only believed to be popular with the kinds of middle-class, 'motivated' parents schools want to attract now but also makes pedagogical sense in the face of tiered assessment regimes and a scarcity of resources. Setting has consequences for the way in which teachers teach and for students' experiences of schooling. The effects of setting on bottom-set students, the difficulties associated with what the EWO at Northwark Park, quoted in the previous chapter, called the creation of a 'D-stream culture' and the tendency for working-class and some groups of black children to be placed in lower sets is well documented (e.g. Oakes 1990; Slavin 1996; Hallam and Toutounji 1996; Boaler 1997a; Sukhnandan and Lee 1998). Boaler's research has also indicated that top-set students, particularly girls, can suffer in a setted environment as well (Boaler 1997b).

---

18 Chapter 5 uses the cases of Ruskin and Beatrice Webb to undertake a more detailed examination of the differential impact on schools of the material and socio-economic contexts within which they are located.

Andrew Martin, a head of year at Ruskin, identified what he perceived to be the negative consequences for bottom-set girls of the introduction of setting in science the previous year in the school. He described a situation in which 'nice girls' were placed in bottom sets with 'a bunch of horrible boys'. Not only were the girls 'turned off science' but their confidence took 'a real knock back . . . It'd be interesting to know if there's a direct link . . . we had four girls who had real confidence problems this year . . . and three of them were taught in those groups'. If Andrew Martin's suspicions are correct and generalisable, then the specific consequences of setting for *girls* have serious ramifications beyond the immediate setted environment.

Mark Foreman had been teaching the 'fast-track' science group at Fletcher School since the reintroduction of setting in the subject the previous year:

Interviewer: Does it change the way you teach, fast track?
M. Foreman: Yeah, you are all doing it at one level, there's much less time for differentiation and much less individual attention to give to the children, because you've got more kids in the group. So yeah, I have felt that I've changed it. I don't like it . . . It's much less small group work, much less individual work with children.

Mark Foreman believes that the tendency towards whole-class teaching associated with setting inculcates a degree of passivity on the part of the less 'able' children in the group:

The bottom third of that group are really struggling. They can see other people doing a lot better than them. They've not got the personal involvement . . . What we've got here is 29 kids in the group, all doing special level work, all on the board, all doing exactly the same thing, and the onus [to do more work] isn't on them. They are in the top set and some of them at the bottom end could take it a bit easy.

The emotional consequences of setting for teachers, particularly those teaching the bottom sets, are profound. As Shirin Kahn, a science teacher at Fletcher, put it, 'It's hell teaching the bottom set, just hell'.

In this last section I have described a shift from what can loosely be characterised as progressive approaches to teaching to more traditional pedagogies. However, some qualification is necessary. I do not want to suggest that English schools, including the ones in our study, were hotbeds of progressive and democratic practice violently disrupted by the imposition of the national curriculum and market forces. During the welfarist era the competitive academic curriculum and its associated pedagogical practices had remained hegemonic in the English school system. More specifically: relatively strong boundaries between subjects were maintained; in practice, the dominant pedagogical approach in the majority of secondary schools continued to be based on a view of teaching as the transmission of knowledge from teacher to pupil and on an individualist conception of learning; and in many schools (particularly in maths and modern languages departments) setting and the regular testing of pupils were the norm. At the same time, however, welfarism did enable pockets of progressivism and innovation to develop and thrive. New subjects, like sociology and media studies, had been introduced and gained status during the period. Streaming was totally abandoned in many schools. And a significant number of teachers felt able and encouraged to employ progressive pedagogies, characterised, for example, by attempts to blur traditional subject boundaries and the use of the students' own backgrounds, experiences and relationships as a major source of curriculum content. Nor do I want to suggest that, where progressive practice exists, it is being wiped out by the PWEPC. John Edwards, the humanities teacher at Ruskin quoted above talking about the new humanities curriculum he constructed, is by no means untypical. What the evidence does indicate, however, is that post-welfarist structures and discourses seem to have produced a climate in schools which is hostile to progressivism. In other words, it would appear to be the case that the John Edwardses of this world are having to work much harder to continue to put their progressivist principles into practice.

Conclusions

My main contention in this chapter has been that the culture of teachers' work is changing in significant ways. In short, teachers are experiencing a loss of autonomy and an accelerated intensification of activity and stress. There is a decline in the sociability of teaching and there is pressure on teachers to adopt more traditional pedagogies, with a focus on output rather than process and on particular groups of higher-attaining students. These effects are produced and embedded within schools by two major 'relay devices', which facilitate state control over teachers and their classroom practices.

   First, there is the change in the availability and distribution of resources to schools inaugurated by the PWEPC – i.e., the shift to *per capita* funding and open enrolment and the competitive local school markets that these mechanisms produce. In this chapter and in Chapter 3 we have seen how funding shortages associated with marketisation can contribute to the adoption of more traditional pedagogies, and how marketisation leads schools and teachers to focus on the kinds of approaches and activities which they think will make them more popular with particular kinds of parents. These are the middle-class parents whose children are the cheapest to teach. Despite research evidence to the contrary (e.g., David *et al.* 1994; Woods *et al.* 1998), school heads and governors appear to believe that such parents are *primarily* concerned about a school's examination league table performance. And so marketisation serves to feed and perpetuate the second major relay device – the discourse of performativity that now pervades schooling and the education system more generally. This discourse represents a way of thinking, talking and acting which gives priority to performance, productivity and output, and which values the measurement of these things as a means of ensuring 'accountability' and 'quality'. As Ball (1999a) defines it:

> Performativity is a technology, a culture and a mode of regulation, or a system of 'terror' in Lyotard's words, that employs judgements, comparisons and displays as means of control, attrition and change. The performances (of individual subjects or organizations) serve as measures of productivity or output, or displays of 'quality', or 'moments' of promotion . . . or inspection. They stand for, encapsulate or represent the worth, quality or value of an individual or organization within a field of judgement.
>
> (Ball 1999a: 2, citing Lyotard 1984)

Performativity contributes to the constitution of new subjectivities whereby teachers 'are represented and encouraged to think about themselves as individuals who calculate about themselves, and "add value" to themselves, improve their productivity, live an existence of calculation' (Ball 1999a: 20). As we have seen in this chapter, the discourse of performativity also undermines teacher autonomy and sociability, and it generates an intensification of the labour process of teaching, a refocusing – and narrowing – of pedagogic activity, and a concomitant shift in who and what is valued in schools. However, I have also alluded to differences in the way these devices impact on teachers. For example, I have suggested that teachers in popular schools with relatively healthy budgets have the most latitude to protect the work that they value. In the following chapter, I want to explore some of these differences in more depth, by looking at how the discursive, material and socio-economic contexts within which schools operate have a differential effect on what school managers and teachers can do.

5 Can all schools be successful?

One of the assumptions underlying post-welfarist educational policies is that in a devolved system of provision so-called failing schools are largely the product of poor leadership and teaching, and that, through the 'cascading of best practice', all schools can be a success. A contrasting view is that good leadership and teaching can only ever have a fairly minimal effect on school performance and that, in trying to locate the source of underperformance, there is a need to focus on factors which are beyond the control of schools, namely social inequality and poverty. It is from this perspective that Peter Robinson (1997: 17) has concluded that 'Over the long run the most powerful educational policy is arguably one which tackles child poverty, rather than any modest interventions in schooling'. This kind of argument is often derided by supporters of markets and managerialism in education, including those in the school improvement camp (e.g., Barber 1996: 131) (see also Chapter 1).

However, some school improvement researchers are careful to emphasise that while schools can and do make a difference, what they can achieve is 'partial and limited, because schools are also part of the wider society, subject to its norms, rules, and influences' (Mortimore 1997: 483). Reynolds and Packer (1992) concluded from their review of school effectiveness research that schools have an independent effect of only 8–15 per cent on student outcomes. And a study by Thomas and Mortimore of the value-added results from one local authority concluded that: 'Once background factors have been accounted for, the variation in pupil's total examination scores attributable to schools is 10 per cent' (Thomas and Mortimore 1996: 26). It is presumably this kind of finding which led Peter Mortimore, an eminent figure in the school improvement community, to join forces with the sociologist Geoff Whitty to challenge the hegemonic belief that it is school managers and teachers who are primarily responsible for educational under-attainment. In particular, Mortimore and Whitty (1997: 8) criticised school improvement work for tending 'to exaggerate the extent to which individual schools can challenge . . . structural inequalities'. Whilst the authors recognised that 'committed and talented heads and teachers can improve schools even if such schools contain a proportion of disadvantaged pupils', they went on to warn 'of the dangers of basing a national strategy for change on the efforts of outstanding individuals working in exceptional circumstances' (Mortimore and Whitty 1997: 6):

> Whilst some schools can succeed against the odds, the possibility of them doing so, year in and year out, still appears remote given that the long-term patterning of educational inequality has been strikingly consistent throughout the history of public education in most countries.
>
> (Mortimore and Whitty 1997: 8–9)

These kind of arguments are relatively commonplace within the sociology of education literature (for example, Angus 1993; Elliot 1996; Hatcher 1998) but it is rare for such arch scepticism about the transformative potential of school improvement strategies to emanate from within the school improvement research community itself. As Martin Thrupp (1998: 98) has argued, while policy makers and school improvers 'may be aware of the influence of social class on student outcomes', there is nevertheless a tendency for them to 'place faith in formal school management, curricula and assessment reforms to bring about changes to student performance'. Thrupp's research indicates that such faith may well be misplaced. He argues that the social mix of schools (what he refers to as the student mix) strongly influences 'school organizational and management processes so as to drag down the academic effectiveness of schools in low SES [socio-economic status] settings and boost it in middle class settings', and concludes that 'schools with differing SES intake compositions will, in fact, not be able to carry out similarly effective school polices and practices even with similar levels of resourcing and after taking account of individual student backgrounds' (Thrupp 1998: 98).

This chapter will attempt to shed light on the issues raised in this often polarised debate around effective schooling by exploring some of the complexities involved in trying to uncover the determinants of the differential 'success' of schools. In doing so, the chapter challenges the oversimplification that characterises many of the arguments around school improvement by demonstrating that it is not a question of *either* management and teaching *or* society determining the success or otherwise of schools. Drawing on qualitative research, the chapter demonstrates the intricate and intimate connections between what school managers and teachers do, and the socio-economic and discursive contexts within which they operate.

The chapter focuses on two inner-London secondary schools, John Ruskin and Beatrice Webb. Both schools are co-educational comprehensive schools but they are very different. Ruskin, which also featured in Chapter 4, is highly regarded within the local community, heavily oversubscribed and performs well in the national league tables of examination results. Beatrice Webb (which featured in Chapters 2 and 4) is located within a mile of Ruskin, has a poor reputation, is very undersubscribed and is positioned near to the bottom of the examination league tables.[19]

I want to begin by briefly sketching out some key background details about the two schools. Then I will explore some of the differences between them in terms of management and teaching, before going on to consider the implications of the schools' social, material and discursive environments for the way in which they operate.

The schools

Ruskin is extremely popular, so much so that students have to live within three-quarters of a mile of the school to gain a place. The intake reflects the social mix of the local area, with approximately a quarter of the children coming from middle-class homes and just over 20 per cent qualifying for free school meals. The intake is mainly white with significant minorities of African-Caribbean, Chinese, Bangladeshi and Indian students. Although 14 per cent come from a home where English is not the first language, the majority of these students were born in Britain and only a handful need extra language support. Fifteen per cent of the students are on the school's register of special educational needs. As is the case with many popular schools, parents have been known to lie about their address in order to secure a place for their children at the school. In 1991 Ruskin expanded its Year 7 intake by 20 per cent in order to accommodate growing demand and to maximise income. Ruskin's examination results are

19 The schools were studied as part of an ESRC–funded project investigating the impact of educational reform on the culture and values of schooling (see Footnote 3 and Appendix).

above the national average. When the research was carried out in 1996, 46 per cent of students got five or more GCSE grades A–C compared to a national average of 45 per cent. The Ofsted team that inspected Ruskin in spring 1996, whilst not uncritical of some aspects of the school, was on the whole highly complimentary, describing it as follows:[20]

> The school aims to provide an environment in which its members can contribute and achieve. It is concerned for the development of the whole person, with learning through personal interest and commitment, with social development through collaboration and shared activity, with exercising choice and self-determination, and with acknowledging rights balanced with responsibilities. Raising achievement is a key objective for which there are planned developments and targets in curriculum planning, managing behaviour and assessment and monitoring. Increased popularity has brought about the opportunity for building development.

Thus, measured against the key public indicators – market performance, examination results and Ofsted report – Ruskin is an unqualified success.

Beatrice Webb, less than a mile away, is markedly undersubscribed and has a poor local reputation. As noted in Chapter 2, very few students choose to go there, the vast majority ending up at the school by default rather than choice. There is a proliferation of short-term accommodation in the area (the chair of governors referred to it as 'bedsit land') and many children enter the school mid-year because their families have been temporarily 'housed' in the area. The school also accepts a significant number of children who have been excluded from other schools. Approximately 35 per cent of the students are refugees, 60 per cent are bi- or multi-lingual and 73 per cent are eligible for free school meals. Thirty per cent of the students are registered as having special educational needs. In January 1996 Beatrice Webb had 520 students on roll, although the school is deemed to have a potential capacity of 900 pupils. It consistently performs poorly in the examination league tables, with nine per cent of students attaining five or more A–C grades at GCSE in 1996.

During the course of the research there was a change of headship at Beatrice Webb, as discussed in Chapter 2. Ofsted inspected the school

---

20 Source details are not supplied for the two Ofsted reports referred to in this chapter in order to protect the anonymity of the schools.

in the spring term of 1996 when the new head had been in the post for under two terms. They concluded that it was a school 'with major weaknesses' and that, although the new head was beginning to tackle these, a lot of work still needed to be done:

> The headteacher was appointed in September 1995 and faced major problems, which, though diminished, still exist. The school was overstaffed, there were grave financial difficulties, standards were low, and the school was heavily undersubscribed. Since his appointment, many beneficial changes have taken place. Although there are still major problems, the school, though it has a long way to go, is slowly improving.

Whilst the inspectors were complimentary about some aspects of the school, they were highly critical of others, pointing in particular to low standards of attainment, poor rates of attendance and punctuality, and a failure of some staff to rigorously 'implement the measures recently undertaken by the school to remedy these deficiencies'.

How do we explain why one of these schools is judged a success and one is considered to be seriously underperforming and in need of being 'turned around'? Clearly, questions need to be asked about the criteria against which success and failure are measured. Success and failure are discursively constructed and we cannot simply take these public discourses at face value. I will return to this issue below, but for the moment, I want to focus on management and teaching in the schools. As I noted at the start of this chapter, a key post-welfarist assumption is that in a devolved system of provision, school managers and teachers are primarily responsible for the success or failure of schools. This assumption gains its legitimacy in part from academic discourses provided by the school effectiveness and improvement lobby (see Chapter 1). In the following section I want to begin to examine the validity of such arguments by comparing teaching and management in Ruskin and Beatrice Webb.

Management and teaching in the two schools

In a review of the school effectiveness literature, Peter Mortimore identifies two research approaches. The first is concerned to isolate the determinants of *successful* schools. Thus, for example, Maden and Hillman (NCE 1995):

emphasize the importance of a cluster of behaviours: a leadership stance which builds on and develops a team approach; a vision of success which includes a view of how the school can improve and which, once it has improved, is replaced by a pride in its achievement; school policies and practices which encourage the planning and setting up of targets; the improvement of the physical environment; common expectations about pupil behaviour and success; and an investment in good relations with parents and the community.

(Mortimore 1997: 481)

The other approach is to identify the causes of school *failure*. For instance, Stoll (1995):

has drawn our attention to lack of vision, unfocused leadership, dysfunctional staff relationships, and ineffective classroom practices as mechanisms through which the effectiveness of schools can deteriorate.

(Mortimore 1997: 481)

So to what extent were any of these features apparent in Ruskin and Beatrice Webb and to what extent can such features be said to *explain* the differential performance of the schools?

Ruskin

Ruskin certainly appears to possess all the features that Maden and Hillman (NCE 1995) associate with successful schools and none of those which Stoll (1995) associates with ineffective schools. The study did not set out to evaluate the teaching in the schools, so for the purposes of reporting on the 'effectiveness' of classroom practice in the schools, I will cite Ofsted's judgements (although these do need to be treated with caution). Ofsted's opinion of teaching at Ruskin was formulated on the basis of observing 225 lessons. The Ofsted team were on the whole positive about the teaching in the school, reporting that:

Teachers work hard to create harmonious relationships in lessons and to provide lessons which contain an interesting variety of activities which largely sustain the interests of students. A good feature of teaching is the way in which subject teachers work with other professionals, parents and outside speakers to provide an interesting and relevant curriculum . . . Lessons are well planned with clear objectives . . . Clear explanations by teachers leave students in no doubt about what they have to do. Teachers are skilful in ascertaining and developing students' understanding through skilful questioning and reformulating their responses.

There were criticisms too, for example, that 'too often teachers over-direct the thinking of the students' and that 'occasionally teachers dominate lessons by talking too much'. But, of the teaching time they observed, they concluded that 90 per cent of lessons were satisfactory, very good or better.

With regard to leadership at Ruskin, a number of teachers I interviewed were critical of the head, viewing him as autocratic and sometimes bullying. However, at the same time, there was a general feeling amongst staff that they were consulted and listened to, even though they were not always happy with the decisions that were made. Whilst the key decisions were made by the senior management team, there were strong lines of communication between management and staff and a significant degree of what appeared to be constructive debate. Complaints and grievances amongst staff did well up but these tended to reach a point at which they were recognised by senior management and dealt with through discussion and compromise. One of the Senior Management Team (SMT), in particular, seems to have adopted an informal role as conduit between staff and management. He spent more time in the staffroom than the other senior managers and picked up on concerns, which were then relayed back to the rest of the SMT, discussed and responded to. Staff meetings were organised by an elected committee of staff and in such a way as to enable teachers to debate issues in the absence of senior management. Staff were also given the opportunity in these meetings to debate with senior management and a minority of teachers were not afraid to challenge publicly the decisions of the SMT. A committee of staff met regularly with senior management to represent staff concerns and to discuss key decisions and policies within the school. Whilst the head clearly saw this group as a useful device for ensuring that management decisions gained legitimacy amongst staff, the members of the group themselves saw it as a means of influencing management decisions in the interests of staff. And from what I observed, the group appeared to be able to use it quite effectively in this way. I witnessed a number of occasions in which senior management revised decisions in the light of staff protest. Although the school was not run along democratic lines, it appeared to have enough democratic-like features to ensure that staff morale was kept at relatively healthy levels.

As regards 'vision', the head and the SMT had a very clear view of what the school stood for. Whilst there were ideological differences and a range of emphases within the staff, there was a generally agreed commitment to offering students a broad and balanced humanistic curriculum within a relatively relaxed and collaborative atmosphere, where children were encouraged to be academically achieving, independent, critical and caring. Target setting and performance monitoring were now firmly entrenched practices within the school, although many staff were opposed to these and were critical of their effects on their pedagogical practice (see Chapter 4).

Beatrice Webb

Whilst Ruskin appears to possess the characteristics that are supposed to produce effective schools, Beatrice Webb seems to have a number of characteristics which are meant to lead to ineffectiveness, although, according to Ofsted, the school was showing signs of 'improvement'. Ofsted concluded that the bulk of teaching at Beatrice Webb was 'satisfactory or better' and a quarter of 'the teaching was good or very good'. However, they also reported, on the basis of the 141 lessons they inspected, that a quarter of the teaching they observed was of poor quality:

> Too many teachers . . . have expectations for the pupils that are too low and weak techniques of assessment. In some subjects . . . the teaching is flawed by poor subject knowledge, the use of unsuitable methods, and the lack of clear aims for lessons.

There was a significant proportion of teachers who had been in the school a long time, were on relatively high salaries and of whom senior managers were critical in terms of their management and, in some cases, teaching skills. One of the younger teachers described this group as the 'old brigade, middle management, who have been here and are established . . . maybe thirteen, fourteen years [and who are] maybe not willing to change their strategies or ideas and [are] costing the school a great deal of money'. He compared these teachers to recent appointees who were more open to change. The interviews revealed many of the staff to be preoccupied with problems of discipline and management, rather than curriculum-related issues.

As reported in Chapter 2, relations between the old head, Susanna English, and the staff had been extremely strained. Using Stoll's (1995) terminology, they could well be described as 'dysfunctional'. Any change the head tried to implement was blocked by a staff which appeared to be dominated by the 'old brigade' of mainly male 'middle managers'. Discussions between staff and management were confrontational and rarely appeared to contribute to changes in school policies or practices. Many of the staff saw Ms English as a poor manager and they were particularly critical of her for regularly 'taking the side' of children whilst, often publicly, undermining teachers, and for not excluding students for serious misdemeanours, like assaulting a teacher. In contrast, at least for a honeymoon period, many believed the new head, Brian Jones, to be a good man-ager, who was variously described as more honest, open and willing to listen than the previous head. Teachers interviewed in his first term in the post argued that he was improving the culture of the school by appearing more appreciative of teachers and by imposing a more disciplined regime on students who previously would:

> go running straight to the head and have a shoulder to cry on, whereas now . . . hopefully, the head won't give them a shoulder to cry on [and] if they've done something serious they'll be booted out for a couple of days . . . If a child needs dealing with, there are now the procedures where you feel comfortable or confi-dent that they will be dealt with in the correct way.
>
> (Young teacher)

Certainly, the exclusion rate increased significantly in Brian Jones' first term of office. The general feeling amongst staff was that the new head was boosting morale:

> He seems to be able to praise people, boost their confidence a bit more, which is much better. I've had more praise in the past year than I've had in the previous thirteen years. He actually notices where good work is going on, good practice, so he seems to have his finger on the pulse much better.
>
> (Head of department)

However, by his second term in office, the new head had begun to implement redundancies and morale once again began to decline. But the Ofsted team, who inspected Beatrice Webb in 1996, was compli-mentary about the head, presenting him as someone who had begun to 'turn the school around', by tackling such problems as 'overstaffing' and the budget deficit, and by replacing the old, rather vague, one-page development plan with a new one detailing 90 points for action.

Both heads at Beatrice Webb had what Maden and Hillman (NCE 1995) describe as 'a vision of success', although there were important aspects of these visions which were very different. As we saw in Chapter 2, Ms English wanted the school to focus on the needs of its *current* constituency, on refugees and students with emotional and behavioural difficulties. She was concerned to improve exam results but she also wanted Beatrice Webb to be a school that involved students in decision making and celebrated difference. Her stance was captured in her vehement opposition to the introduction of school uniform, which she saw as a means of controlling children by:

> taking away a whole area of choice from kids . . . The variety of clothing that you observe when you go there is quite amazing and I think quite delightful, it's part of that general . . . sense of difference . . . and variety that goes on there.
>
> (Ms English)

Brian Jones' vision, which was more popular with the majority of staff, was to make the school into an institution that would attract a different (more middle-class) constituency and make it a success in market terms. His vision was couched in the language of improvement, and emphasised achievement and discipline whilst downplaying the school's work with refugees. Significantly, his position on uniform was in stark contrast to Ms English's. Whilst she had delighted in the students' varied and expressive responses to the school's liberal dress code, Mr Jones was highly critical. He felt that the lack of uniform contributed to what he described as a holiday camp atmosphere, which was simply not appropriate for an institution that needed to establish itself as a place of learning.

One conclusion that could be drawn from much of the preceding description of teaching and management at the two schools is that the school effectiveness researchers are accurate in their analysis of the determinants of school success and failure. After all, Ruskin could well be described as having:

> a leadership stance which builds on and develops a team approach; a vision of success which includes a view of how the school can improve . . . school policies and practices which encourage the planning and setting up of targets; the improvement of the physical

environment; common expectations about pupil behaviour and success; and an investment in good relations with parents and the community.

(Mortimore 1997: 481)

And all of these things might be said to account for why Ruskin performs so well according to public indicators. Equally, Beatrice Webb's 'underperformance' could be attributed to a number of past failures, in particular: the absence of a team approach to school management; a failure to develop a vision of success couched in the language of improvement; a neglect of planning and target-setting practices; a neglect of the physical environment; 'dysfunctional' staff relationships and a lack of agreement between staff and management around expectations of pupil behaviour; and ineffective classroom practices. If we are to accept Ofsted's assessment, then we might predict that the new head's attempts to try and rectify some of the weaknesses will lead to improved performance at Beatrice Webb.

However, whilst there may well be a *correlation* between particular features of management and teaching and degrees of school success, we need to be a little wary of concluding that the relationship is *causal* or at least we should not assume that it is causal in the direction that school effectiveness researchers claim it is. In the next section, I want to delve a little deeper and explore some of the features of the social environments of the two schools that might account for the differences between them in terms of management and teaching.

The impact of social environment

Drawing upon an ethnographic study of four New Zealand schools, Martin Thrupp very convincingly demonstrates the 'stubborn constraints on organizational and management processes in low SES [socio-economic status] schools compared to their middle-class counterparts' (1998: 216). In particular, he identifies 'intense pressures on teachers and school leaders generated by students in low SES schools' (1998: 214). As a result of these pressures, Thrupp concludes, 'time and energy required to consider and implement demands from central agencies will be scarce in low SES schools'. In addition, he argues that 'teachers and principals at (low SES) declining schools are so overwhelmed with pastoral and learning problems that they will be unable to deliver similar academic programmes as middle class schools' (1998: 214–15).

An analysis of the impact of student demands on management and teaching processes at Ruskin and Beatrice Webb would appear to support Thrupp's conclusions about the importance of social mix in determining the 'success' of schools. There are a number of features of Beatrice Webb's intake that create particular demands for the staff. Some of the English as an additional language speakers come to the school with poor levels of literacy in their first language. As well as the challenge of having to learn a new language, many of the refugee students have emotional difficulties linked to experiences of war in their countries of origin, moving to a strange country and living in bed-and-breakfast accommodation, or arriving without parents and having to settle into local authority care.

In addition, Beatrice Webb has a highly mobile population, in part because the community the school serves is highly transient and in part because many of the students who enter the school in Year 7 are on waiting lists for their first choice schools. When a vacancy in one of those schools comes up, the student will leave, and such departures can occur even when a student has reached Year 10. The head of Year 7 at Beatrice Webb noted that many of the students who were offered places at other schools were higher attaining students who would have enhanced the school's league table performance had they remained in the school until Year 11. At the same time, there were students, across the age spectrum, who joined the school regularly throughout the school year, either because they had been excluded from other schools or because they had been moved into short-term housing of which there is a considerable quantity in the vicinity of the school. One of the younger teachers in the school defined the problem and the difficulties it creates in the following way:

> Because we are so skint, we need money and we tend to accept any-body who comes along. So . . . we lose our best kids to the other schools, because waiting lists are freed up and they've got spare places . . . and in exchange we get kids who have been excluded from those schools who often are the rather unfriendly ones who are aggressive and have been excluded for bad reasons. And we then have to deal with them. So throughout the year . . . there is literally a twenty per cent change in pupils in each year. And only about twenty per cent actually manage to make it through the first year to the fifth year. So you've got different faces all the time. Even in Year 11 you are getting different faces, which makes it very difficult to teach and later in the year you get the worst pupils. We start off with some very nice ones but then lose

them to other schools, because nobody picks Beatrice Webb as a first choice, which is a shame.

A highly mobile population can create a number of quite difficult challenges for teachers. Teachers have to establish relationships with new students on a weekly basis. They have to settle these students into their classes, induct them into their particular teaching styles, assess the students' abilities, learning styles, language skills and what, if anything, they have already covered in the curriculum. In addition, the composition of classes constantly changes, which in itself can be disruptive, as one head of department explained:

> It makes it very difficult, not just for teaching, as in trying to cover all the work that these children should have done in the past, because they arrive with no records, especially if they're refugees, but also in terms of [the] socio dynamics of the group, in that a group can be quite settled and get a new student every fortnight, and it will just disrupt the whole group dynamic . . . and a group that would have been settled and working well, can become then a very difficult group to teach, because of shifting pressures within the group.

And finally, many of the new arrivals, having been excluded from other schools, can exhibit challenging forms of behaviour. According to one of the teachers interviewed, many of the children excluded from other schools succeed at Beatrice Webb and he put this down to the school ethos:

> It's not a regimented strongly disciplinarian place . . . there's an atmosphere which is about groups, about caring for each other . . . it's a very good atmosphere.
>
> (Language support teacher)

The Ofsted team made a similar observation about the quality of relationships between and amongst staff and students in the school:

> Most pupils and teachers like and respect each other. Pupils come from widely differing backgrounds and nationalities, and are tolerant towards each other. No direct evidence of bullying was found . . . Many pupils show concern for other newly arrived pupils or for those whose English is limited. There are many instances of pupils helping others in lessons.

However, it was the general consensus in the school that a small minority of students who had been excluded from at least one other school – some were 'serial excludees' – were an extremely disruptive influence, taking up a disproportionate quantity of teacher and management time. The headteacher had to deal on a daily basis with violent episodes involving these few students. Incidents occurring in the school during a typical two months of the fieldwork period included students attacking each other with a police baton, bottles, a baseball bat and an airgun. One of these episodes was connected to a drug-related dispute. Dealing with these incidents was immensely time consuming, involving liaising variously with teachers, students, parents (of both perpetrators and victims), the police and social workers. If the head wanted to exclude the culprits, then he needed to be meticulous in his collection of evidence by interviewing student witnesses and in recording that evidence.

Ruskin was not free of violence and student conflict but there was not nearly as much of it. Because Ruskin is full, it does not need to accept any excluded students. When it has a vacancy, it can take a student from its long waiting list. These students tend to be the ones that Beatrice Webb and other local schools would like to retain. Harvey Smith, a head of year at Ruskin, commented that the students the school accepted when there was a vacancy tended to be very motivated high achievers:

> I could name probably nine or ten kids, we've taken them from Winbrook [a nearby school] and every one of them's been a diamond, you know. They've all been really good . . . and they've been academic, hardworking kids. We haven't taken any bad kids from Winbrook . . . they're all cracking kids . . . And there's probably ten who've come into Year 10, you know, since they've come in perhaps in Year 7 or 8, 9, 10. We take them from other schools as well . . . But we don't take bad kids . . . *And we are doing well at the expense of other schools.*
>
> (My italics)

Focusing on the impact of student mix should not be seen as an exercise in pathologising the students in working-class schools or of blaming them for schools' weaknesses but school populations have different needs and create different demands, which need to be acknowledged. Teachers in schools like Beatrice Webb need very special skills to deal with the challenges thrown up by their intakes and at Beatrice

Webb there were simply not enough specialists. For example, the school had a total of three and a half specialist language support teachers. These were allocated to different faculties: English was the most 'generously' resourced with the equivalent of one full-time and one part-time teacher, science had a full-time teacher and geography and technology shared a support teacher. This left 'history uncovered . . . [and] maths gets a raw deal' (language support teacher). One of the science teachers we interviewed did not have any language support teachers in any of the classes he taught. A language support teacher explained the difficulties involved in teaching classes with a high proportion of students classified as 'stage one' learners (i.e., those who are just beginning to learn to speak and write in English):

> There are subjects which have no support at all, and [it is] very difficult [for one teacher] to organise a classroom when there are perhaps four or five who can't read at all, very difficult, and then all the difficulties of . . . if the text is very complicated, how does everyone understand them, how do you access the understanding . . . so part of that is to introduce ways of doing that, perhaps providing lists of words, glossaries, cutting up the text into more manageable sections, but . . . it takes so long to actually devise stuff, you can't, as a normal mainstream teacher, you can't be expected to do that. I think you are expected, but in terms of time, you don't have time.

However, it is not just a question of time for curriculum planning and the production of learning support materials. There is also considerable skill involved in making the curriculum accessible to a diverse range of stage one learners. Many of the teachers who had not had specialist training in fact did very well. To take a crude indicator, GCSE results in art and drama were well above the national average for comprehensive schools. However, it was noticeable that the staff and departments which performed particularly well in external examinations were from those subjects in which students were less dependent on literacy skills for success. This is not to detract from the talent of the teachers in these departments but it may well be that these subjects are more accessible to students not yet fluent in English.

The pressures generated by the student mix at Beatrice Webb also meant it was much harder for teachers to channel energy into extra-curricular activities. And take up of extra-curricular opportunities was much lower at Beatrice Webb than at Ruskin, possibly because students had greater domestic responsibilities, for example, caring for younger siblings or helping their parents, for instance as interpreters, in ways which Ruskin students did not have to. Ofsted noted that 'school concerts, performances and musical activities are rare' at Beatrice Webb.

Ofsted were generally positive about the teaching of refugee students and those with special needs at Beatrice Webb, leading them to conclude that:

> Given the very mixed nature of the school's intake, satisfactory progress is being made by about 70 per cent of the pupils. The school has a good and justified reputation for providing well for non-indigenous and refugee children, who generally make satisfactory progress. Such progress is also made by pupils with special educational needs, who are well catered for throughout the school.

They also noted that in three subject areas there was good practice in marking, record keeping and assessment, and they noted 'several examples of first rate team teaching . . . with the support and the class teacher each sharing the lead and making full use of their skills'.

But it is unsurprising that a significant minority of teachers at Beatrice Webb could not cope with the pressures exerted upon them and could not adequately perform all of the tasks now expected of teachers. A trained observer might well view these teachers as less than competent but it is possible that if these same teachers were teaching in schools with a less challenging student mix, they would be judged satisfactory. Charlene Fraser, a languages teacher at Ruskin, had previously taught at another local school, Applegate, which was very similar to Beatrice Webb in terms of its intake. She commented that there were many staff at Ruskin 'who would not be able to teach at Applegate, and they recognise that and that's why they wouldn't be at that sort of school'. She also described the sheer physicality and emotionality of teaching in a school like Applegate, where behavioural concerns tend to overshadow curricular ones:

> You are not as physically tired at the end of the day working in this sort of school [Ruskin], because . . . your classroom doesn't have to be managed in quite such [a] physical way, and the children don't demand as much of you in this sort of school . . . Because the children there [at Applegate] have so little – a lot of the children don't have much input from parents – they're very, very demanding.

Charlene went on to argue that at Ruskin the lack of physicality involved in the work and the fact that the children were less demanding meant that more emphasis could be placed on reflecting upon and refining the curriculum:

> The emphasis on the curriculum here [at Ruskin] is paramount, because behaviour problems don't get in the way in the same way that they do at Applegate . . . And the importance at Applegate is really to create an atmosphere in which work can be done and in which the children feel safe and secure . . . with the curriculum obviously running alongside. And that's what . . . makes it very difficult at that school. Whereas here the curriculum is really what . . . we're always changing and pushing forward . . . We're really looking at the curriculum all the time. [We] spend very little time, really, worrying about disciplining classes.

Charlene also described how a less demanding intake makes the management of a school and the development of constructive and collaborative relationships easier:

> It's easier to make something work, like an ideal plan of management, a structure, if you don't have a lot of other issues that really get in the way and hijack agendas . . . I feel that at Applegate what happened was that there would be issues which would hijack agendas constantly . . . And because . . . there was conflict in the community so therefore there was a certain amount of conflict within how we thought it should be managed . . . [Whereas at Ruskin] where things are seen to work pretty well, although we have our gripes and things, there isn't a lot of conflict between management and us really.

Charlene was making some important and astute points here and her analysis of the way in which agendas were hijacked at Applegate and of the conflict generated by the social environment of the school applies equally to Beatrice Webb. The head at Ruskin had time to devote himself to strategic issues and the budget. Much of the day-to-day running of the school was delegated to the deputies, senior teachers and heads of department and year. On occasion, the head had to deal with student disciplinary matters and complaining parents but rarely was a whole day taken up with dealing with a crisis caused by, say, an episode of student violence. And, as Charlene was arguing, because things were seen to work well at Ruskin, morale was relatively healthy and serious conflict between staff and management did not arise.

At Beatrice Webb, Brian Jones probably needed more time for strategic planning than the head of Ruskin because the problems the school faced were so much more profound – severe under-recruitment, a poor local reputation, the huge budget deficit, the underfunding of departments, poor relations between management and staff and a highly demanding student population. But in fact he had much less time for planning than the head of Ruskin. Both Ms English and Mr Jones invested an enormous amount of energy and time into dealing with violent and/or disruptive students and, unlike the head of Ruskin, they found it difficult to free themselves from the day-to-day running of the school in order to focus on strategic planning and to develop initiatives that might have improved recruitment. For example, one of Mr Jones' first initiatives when he joined the school in 1995 was a club for 10–12 year olds, which was designed to try and get more primary age students into the school and cultivate them as potential recruits. But by 1997 this had still not got off the ground, simply because the SMT's time was taken up with more pressing day-to-day activities. In addition, because the work of teaching is so much more demanding at Beatrice Webb, because of the intractability of many of the problems the school faces and because of the budget deficit and the fear of redundancy, morale was extremely low. This undoubtedly created tension in the school and must have exacerbated, if not produced, the bitterly conflictual relationships that existed between managers and staff in the school.

Furthermore, the relatively harmonious relationships at Ruskin, and the latitude that teachers had to focus on the curriculum and to practice relatively progressive pedagogies, contributed to its reputation as a good school in which to work. It was also a growing school and, as a result of these things, it was able to attract talented, dynamic and committed teachers. By contrast, Beatrice Webb was a school which was making redundancies and, although it did have its share of highly skilled and imaginative staff, there was, according to some of the more recent recruits, a significant minority of disillusioned and cynical teachers who had lost the energy to be creative. It is much harder to attract 'good' teachers to a school which is conflict-ridden, under-resourced and with low morale.

Another feature of the social environment that makes managing a more middle-class school easier is the higher levels of parental involvement and the fact that parents are more accessible in more middle-class schools. Ruskin had an active parents' association and the annual governors' meeting for parents was well-attended. The SMT did not need to invest a lot of energy into developing relationships with parents. If anything, they had the opposite problem – many parents who wanted to be involved with the nitty gritty of classroom practice, for example, the finer points of teaching grammar in French lessons. In addition, Ruskin had a highly skilled and involved governing body with high levels of cultural capital. For example, one of the parent governors was a very senior civil servant and another the principal of a further education college.

At Beatrice Webb, attempts were made to develop relations with parents through the appointment, under Ms English, of a deputy head responsible for community relations but promoting parental and community involvement proved difficult. There was no parents' association at Beatrice Webb, very few parents ever attended the governing body's annual report meeting for parents (only the parent governors attended in 1994 and in 1995 only one parent who was not a governor turned up – and the chair of governors commented that this parent only 'came along . . . to have something to do, if even to get out of the bloody horrible hotel' (where she had been temporarily accommodated by the LEA)). Only five parents attended the pre-inspection meeting held by the Ofsted Registered Inspector and just seven (1.4 per cent) of the 500 questionnaires for parents that Ofsted sent out were returned. (This compared with a response rate of 29 per cent at Ruskin.) Furthermore, the governors at Beatrice Webb were not skilled at reading and scrutinising budgets like those at Ruskin, and they did not contribute the same levels of support, for example, by visiting departments within the school, although strenuous efforts had been made to involve them more.

The material environment

It was not just the social mix but the material environment at Beatrice Webb which made it a more difficult place than Ruskin in which to work. In fact, Beatrice Webb spent more per student than did Ruskin (£3,400 was spent at Beatrice Webb per student in 1995–96 compared with £2,500 at Ruskin). However, this was probably mainly because the overheads at Beatrice Webb (i.e., heating, maintenance and ensuring adequate curriculum coverage) constituted a higher proportion of expenditure than at Ruskin because the school had an intake of less than half the size. Yet far more resources are needed for a population of the kind that characterises Beatrice Webb. The school needs more in-class support and more materials to support second language learners and students with special needs. In the 1995–96 school year, the language support department at Beatrice Webb spent its entire annual photocopying budget by Christmas and was forced to resort to getting the old Gestetner machine working again. During the same school year, the science department had an annual budget of £4.46 per student, which was £3.50 less than any other school in the authority. The department had to choose between photocopying differentiated materials, buying chemicals or buying paper or exercise books. There is little scope for eliciting funds from parents, the majority of whom are on income support, and one of the teachers we interviewed told us that he often subsidises school trips and other activities 'out of my pocket, rather than the school funds, and I suspect I'm not the only teacher in the school that does this' (Steve Davis, head of department).

One could argue that the insufficiency of resources was the result of a failure of management to bring in more money into the school, and there is some truth to this. Language support money is not part of the LMS budget and is subject to a separate bidding system within the local authority. One of the support teachers noted that the previous school he worked in, which was in the same authority, had twice as many support teachers although not as many stage one learners. He suggested that the reason for this was that the senior managers at his previous school exhibited more skill in the bidding process. This raises the question of whether a bidding system is the fairest and most rational way to allocate resources for essential services like language support (see Chapter 8).

Beatrice Webb was technically overstaffed because it had a higher teacher-student ratio than was deemed appropriate (with 13 students per qualified teacher compared to 15 at Ruskin) and as a result redundancies were being made. At the same time it had larger class sizes, with an average teaching group size of 24, compared with 22 at Ruskin. Now again, the larger classes in a school with more teachers could be attributed to poor management of resources. However, not only did Beatrice Webb need to ensure that it covered the same subject areas as Ruskin but the teachers also needed more planning time – for subject teachers to liaise with language and learning support teachers about how best to meet the curriculum needs of the students and because of the relatively high level of demand for pastoral support.

The physical condition of the school also made a difference in terms of teaching and learning. Whilst Ruskin was not lavishly decorated and furnished, and more improvements were needed, the internal and external environment was pleasant and had been recently subjected to a programme of development. At Beatrice Webb, the situation was very different. Ofsted noted the poor physical condition of the school, commenting (accurately) that:

> While the accommodation is adequate overall, much of it is poorly maintained and in need of refurbishment. Classrooms are in need of decoration and much of the furniture, though adequate, is of poor quality. The classroom environment is often uninviting and unconducive to the production of high quality work. Classrooms for English have poor blackboard surfaces, from which it is difficult to read, and the rooms would benefit greatly by the provision of whiteboards. Science laboratories have no blinds, which prevent certain experiments being carried out. Changing rooms for physical education are inadequate and the gyms are often dirty, corridors are in need of decoration and, where carpets are provided, they are often badly stained.

The importance of material resources for school 'success' has been highlighted by a set of case studies published by the DFEE (1997a), which describe some of the ways improvement has been achieved in schools that have failed their Ofsted inspections. Mortimore and Whitty conclude from these studies that: 'In contrast to much of the rhetoric about resources not mattering, what stands out is the impact of the extra resources invested by the LEAs in their efforts to turn the schools round' (1997: 6). Mortimore and Whitty also cite the work of Barbara MacGilchrist (1997) who concludes from a review of research on the links between disadvantage and achievement that considerable financial investment is needed if interventions to raise reading attainment of students from 'disadvantaged' backgrounds are to be successful.

Performativity and market discourses

A third environmental factor is the discourses of performativity and markets that now surround and permeate education provision (see Chapter 4). It is these discourses which have constructed Beatrice Webb as a failure and Ruskin as a success. Ruskin is a success because its students are seen to perform well in national tests and examinations, because it is popular with parents and because Ofsted says it is good. Beatrice Webb, on the other hand, is a failure because its students are not considered to perform well in tests, it is undersubscribed and Ofsted found major weaknesses.

These discourses and the criteria of success/failure embedded within them were internalised within the schools. For example, at Beatrice Webb some of the governors were critical of the school because of the low percentage of students getting five or more A–C grades at GCSE. And at both schools, teaching was increasingly focused upon raising levels of performance in GCSEs and SATs, and in particular on those students likely to get C grades and above (see Chapter 4). But the discourses were also challenged in both schools, and particularly at Beatrice Webb where they were viewed as highly inappropriate. For example, one of the science teachers at Beatrice Webb commented:

> I know there are some students that I teach in Year 11 who are not going to get graded. It's not because they are not nice kids, it's not because they don't come to school, it's just because their language isn't up to it at present.

And one of the language support teachers argued:

> In the press it's always, the criteria is A to C and therefore the league tables are weighted against schools which are actually achieving, but what they are achieving is not being recognised as an achievement . . . [for] example, someone who comes from Ethiopia in Year 11, say in October, will not have the projects from the first year of the GCSE course and therefore will have to work twice as hard to catch up and also get through the current coursework and then through the exam and learning English at the same time, will have to work so hard to just get, what, an E in the GCSE . . . In geography we're actually thinking that a couple of girls from Ethiopia will get E, maybe even D/Cs . . . It's because they work so hard, they're in local authority homes and therefore for them school is so important, it's the one place which is like secure, where they know people and people are working, helping them.

This teacher was making two important points here. One was that in terms of exam performance, Beatrice Webb was actually doing well for its students, but in a way that was not acknowledged by the public indicators which focus on higher attaining students. Given that students were joining the school with low levels of prior attainment, and also given that many of the higher attaining students were leaving before Year 11, 10 per cent of students getting five or more A–Cs may well have been very good on a value-added calculation. In fact, the statistics indicate that students who had been at the school from Year 7 to Year 11 tended to do well in their GCSEs. But also, simply getting a student who has just come to the country with no prior knowledge of the English language through a GCSE is a major achievement. The other important issue that the language support teacher was drawing our attention to was the fact that there were other aspects of what the school had to offer, which were not being valued by the discourses of the market and performativity – in particular, the provision of a secure and supportive environment for children who have been uprooted from their families and countries of origin and living in an unfamiliar country in difficult circumstances.

Conclusions

In conclusion, I want to highlight some key issues that have emerged from my discussion of the cases of Beatrice Webb and John Ruskin. The first set of issues relates to the discursively constructed nature of effectiveness. I have argued that the discourses of performativity and markets construct schools like Beatrice Webb as failures even though they may be offering very positive experiences, intellectually and socially, for many of their students. What also needs to be emphasised is that hegemonic constructions of effectiveness affect life in schools in quite deep-seated ways. For example, schools constructed as failing suffer poor morale as a consequence. In addition, they are pressed into introducing changes, for example, the use of more didactic teaching methods, which may not be in the best interests of the majority of students attending the schools (see Chapter 4).

The second related set of issues revolves around the complexity of the relationship between school 'effectiveness', management and teaching in schools and the social and material contexts of schooling. The analysis presented in this chapter would seem to suggest that poor performance of schools in exams and in Ofsted inspections and under-subscription correlate with the kinds of features that the school improvement literature associates with failing schools, and that, conversely school 'success' correlates with 'good' management and 'good' teaching. But the chapter has also indicated that one cannot reasonably conclude from this that 'good' management and teaching, are *responsible* for school 'success'. In fact, if the evidence presented here is representative (and obviously more studies of this kind are needed) then it would appear to suggest that the opposite is true: that school 'success' contributes to 'good' management and teaching, and school 'failure' contributes to less 'effective' management and teaching. This is because schools deemed to be successful are likely to have a significant proportion – what Thrupp (1998) refers to as a critical mass – of high attaining and relatively undemanding pupils, they are adequately resourced and can attract talented teachers. As a result of these things, morale is relatively high and teachers can focus their attention on developing imaginative curricula. In 'failing' schools, teachers and managers find that, in the words of one of our informants, the agenda tends to get hijacked by behavioural and resource-related issues. In addition, the students demand more of teachers physically, emotionally and intellectually. And as a result, morale is likely to be low, relationships conflictual and teachers are left with little energy and insufficient resources to develop appropriate and imaginative schemes of work, classroom materials and pedagogical practices.

All of this is not to say that good management and teaching do not make a difference or that it is the nature of catchment areas alone which determines the effectiveness of schools. Rather, what I have tried to illustrate is how the various factors that are normally viewed as contributing to effective schools are bound up with each other in complex ways, and that what managers and teachers do in schools is necessarily heavily influenced by the socio-economic and discursive environments within which they are located. In short, 'internal', school-based determinants of 'success', do not operate independently of 'external', context-based determinants – and any analysis of 'effective' schooling that does not recognise this must be regarded as deeply flawed.

Given the importance of 'external' factors, a logical response for managers of 'unsuccessful' schools is to try and alter the material and social conditions within which they operate by increasing the size and changing the class composition of their student intakes (see Chapters 2 and 3). Research (for example, Gewirtz *et al.* 1995; Hughes and Lauder 1999) and the experience of Beatrice Webb indicate that one of the major criteria for parental choice of schools is class-based; that is, parents choose on the basis of student mix. Beatrice Webb was unlikely ever to be popular with its reputation for violence (because of a tiny minority of violent students) and its intake of mainly working-class students, refugees and bilingual speakers. Local primary headteachers had told the teacher responsible for primary liaison, that some parents *rejected* the school because of its 'very good reputation for being welcoming and helping all sorts of refugee kids'. The primary liaison teacher commented that this 'became the overwhelming view of us and some parents thought the kids might suffer'. The general consensus in the school was that, for Beatrice Webb to improve:

> what we've got to do is attract some middle-class kids and improve the exam results and improve the image of the school and then through that it's a circle that will attract more. It's getting that first kick start, I think.
>
> (Paul McIntosh, head of department)

Whilst the new head Mr. Jones was redistributing resources within the school and targeting them on the needs of the bilingual students, for example, by establishing a reading room and a weekly reading hour, he was also channelling energy into trying to change the social mix of the school. In contrast to his predecessor who had celebrated and given a high profile to the school's refugee work, the new head, as was noted in Chapter 2, made a conscious decision to play down the work of the school in supporting refugees and he introduced uniform as one strategy for persuading middle-class parents to choose the school. Evidence that his efforts were meeting with some success was a letter circulated by a local group of middle-class parents of Year 6 (top-year primary) students appealing to other parents to support and work to improve Beatrice Webb, their local secondary school, by sending their children there.

In the long run, this strategy could conceivably be successful, transforming the social mix of the school by introducing more middle-class, monolingual students, until it is oversubscribed, enabling it to 'improve' according to official indicators so that it is deemed publicly to be a successful school. But if it is to become oversubscribed it will no longer have space for casual entrants, including refugees, who have in the past, according to a number of observers, including Ofsted, been so well-served by the school, and for students with behavioural difficulties who have been excluded from other schools. It will also be attracting middle-class students who would have attended other local schools, possibly creating vacancies in those schools to be filled by the casual entrants who would previously have gone to Beatrice Webb. There is a possibility, therefore, that whilst the fortunes of Beatrice Webb may go up, another school may embark on a downward spiral of market failure and reputational decline, and excluded students will continue to be shunted from school to school.

It would, therefore, appear that *in practice* within a post-welfarist environment, where schooling is governed by the discourses and technologies of the market and performativity, 'good management' is in large part defined as the ability to transform the socio-economic and linguistic make-up of a school. Thus, within the context of the market and a performance-oriented educational system, management, I would suggest, is severely limited because what it is effectively doing is producing a redistribution of students amongst schools. It cannot address the root causes of educational underattainment.

Part II

Assessing post-welfarism in education

6 The post-welfarist settlement in education

Consequences and contradictions

Part I of this book has focused on what has happened inside schools as a consequence of educational post-welfarism. This has involved explorations of: the language and practices of school management; some of the value conflicts with which teachers have had to engage; changes in teachers' activities and subjectivities; the shifting nature of social relations in schools; and the nature of the relationship between what teachers and managers do and the social, material, and discursive contexts within which schools are located. In this part of the book I want to build upon these explorations to identify and make an assessment of the broader sets of trends and tensions associated with post-welfarist policies in education. I begin this task in this chapter by distilling from the analysis in Part I what might be viewed as the defining features of post-welfarism in education and I consider the implications of post-welfarist policies for the problems of the state they were designed to solve. I will go on in Chapter 7 to examine in some detail the implications of post-welfarism for patterns of justice in and around schooling. Finally, in Chapter 8, I will critically examine new Labour's 'third way' for education, focusing on its contradictions and likely consequences.

Defining features of educational post-welfarism

In the introduction to this book (Chapter 1), I argued that educational post-welfarism emerged out of a range of somewhat disparate policies introduced by successive Conservative governments between 1980 and 1997. In the language of state theory, these policies have produced a newly 'stabilised and sedimented set of state structures, practices and modes of calculation' and a new 'articulation of institutional relationships and responsibilities' (Hay 1996: 44). In other words, the policies have effected a restructuring of the relationship between the state and educational institutions, contributing to the establishment of a new educational settlement to supersede the previous welfarist settlement. Most crucially, the policies have effected a shift from a situation in which schools and teachers had a 'licensed autonomy' from the state and the economy to one of 'regulated autonomy' (Dale 1989) in which the state controls the work of schools and teachers through the mechanisms of a highly regulated market and new managerial modes of control, and by creating systems of accountability, inspection and performance monitoring which 'steer' actions and decisions towards targets and set goals. Whilst these mechanisms have effectively produced a tightening of control of teachers' work by the central state, they are somewhat paradoxically anchored in discourses of devolution and decentralisation. Throughout the book I have referred to the range of policies which set these new institutional relationships, values and practices of regulation in train as the post-welfarist education policy complex (PWEPC).

However, in order to understand fully the nature of any settlement and the contradictions arising from it, it is not enough to focus on the *formal structures of regulation* but to consider the cultural, relational and values dimensions of *lived settlements*. The *lived educational post-welfarist settlement* is complex. In Part I of this book I have attempted to capture difference and nuance in the responses of schools. In doing so, I have tried to demonstrate some of the ways in which the shift from welfarism to post-welfarism is complicated and contested. As I argued in Chapter 1, 'welfarism' and 'post-welfarism' are convenient labels, usefully capturing broad shifts in the organisation of welfare and education provision. However, we need to be wary of allowing the use of these labels to let us slip into making crude generalisations about, and comparisons between, the era that can be loosely categorised as welfarist and that which can be loosely categorised as post-welfarist. As we have seen in Part I, in struggling to cope with and make sense of the new policy environment in which they find themselves, individual teachers and headteachers combine, in complicated and diverse ways, languages, practices, values and ways of thinking drawn from both welfarist and post-welfarist discursive repertoires. More specifically, my examination of the shifting discourses of school headship in Chapter 2 demonstrated how the personal ideologies of headteachers and the micro-politics of schools can influence the ways in which school managers interpret and respond to the new legislative framework. And the discussion of 'values drift' in Chapter 3 drew attention to differences in the ways in which governors and teachers actively position themselves in relation to the disciplinary framework imposed by post-welfarist policies. There is clearly still some scope for contestation, although, as the analysis in Chapter 5 indicated, schools working in different socio-economic and material contexts are differentially positioned by the discourses of performativity and the market that now dominates. These different positionings mean that possibilities of flexibility or freedom of manoeuvre are more available to some headteachers, teachers and governors than others.

We also need to be wary of falling into the trap of golden-ageism – of unduly romanticising about the welfarist era in education, which, as Whitty and his colleagues remind us, was 'fundamentally patriarchal and racially structured in its organizing principles and practices' (Whitty *et al.* 1998: 55, citing Williams 1991). There is no doubt that for many black and working-class students, their experience of welfarist education policies was of being consigned to lower ability sets and under-resourced schools and of being stereotyped as low achievers. Even so-called progressive education would have been experienced by many as being patronising and damaging to self-esteem. We need to remember that it was the failure of welfarist policies to meet the expectations of diverse and subordinated social groups which contributed to the problem of legitimation that I have argued post-welfarist policies were, at least in part, designed to solve.

However, having warned against the twin dangers of over-generalisation and romanticisation, I do want to argue that it is possible to distil from the analysis presented in Part I key consequences of the PWEPC which may be said to constitute the defining features of post-welfarist schooling. In Chapter 1, I argued that I wanted to attend to what Michael Apple has referred to as the task of simultaneity, of 'thinking neo and post together', and it is perhaps worth reiterating Apple's concerns about post-structuralist tendencies within the academy at this point. 'There is a world of difference', Apple (1996a: 141) writes, 'between emphasizing the local, the contingent and non-correspondence and ignoring any determinacy or any structural relationships among practices'. Thus, whilst it is important to recognise difference and nuance if we want to accurately capture what is happening in schools as a consequence of post-welfarism, it is nevertheless vital that we do not underestimate the structural and ideological constraints set by the material, social and discursive formations of post welfarism. It is within and against these constraints that the different responses of diverse social agents are articulated. The research reported in Part I suggests that the discursive formations of post-welfarism can produce very distinct effects. In what follows, I discuss these under the following headings:

- the insertion into schools of managerial regimes of regulation
- the commodification and differential valuing of children
- a reconfiguration of the social relations of schooling through the subjugation of classroom teachers and the inculcation of competitive individualism
- the privileging of traditionalist pedagogic regimes
- the exacerbation of inequalities of access to schooling and heightened social stratification
- the penetration into schooling of capitalist values and a capitalist mode of rationality
- the silencing of dissenting voices
- the inculcation of systemic stress.

Of course, in reality, and as will become apparent in the discussion below, these are not distinct features: they overlap and they shape and inform each other. For instance, managerial regimes of regulation help promote the differential valuing of children and their commodification, they reconfigure social relations, they privilege traditional pedagogic regimes, they produce inequality and stratification, they contribute to the silencing of dissenting voices, and they both represent and produce values drift. All of these things in turn contribute to the production of systemic stress. However, it is useful for heuristic purposes to separate these effects out into distinct categories, as follows.

The insertion of new managerial regimes of regulation

In Chapter 2, I suggested that the PWEPC has constructed a new managerial discourse of headship in schools, characterised by shifts in focus, style, practices and language. Heads now have to ensure that their institutions are consumer-responsive. In particular, they may find themselves having to be especially sensitive to the perceived demands of middle-class consumers whose children have become valued commodities in these new times (as long as they do not have special educational needs or exhibit 'behavioural problems'); headteachers have to ensure that their institutions retain or develop a competitive edge over other local schools; they have to manage their budget efficiently and cost-effectively; they have to make decisions about the appointment, utilisation and dismissal of staff, and the purchase and use of physical resources; and they have to try and manage the conflict and dissent produced by the PWEPC.

The PWEPC demands the realignment of school practices to performance criteria set by the state and the new managerialism is the device –
the mode of coordination (see Chapter 1) – which has evolved to effect
this realignment, in particular through the strategies of target-setting,
performance monitoring and a closer surveillance of teachers.

The new managerialism fuses neo-Taylorist management practices
with post-Taylorist ones: in effect it is a composite of old and relatively
new forms of management. Thus, on the one hand, policy formulation
and policy execution are becoming distinct practices within schools,
with senior managers developing policy in line with the requirements
of the PWEPC and teachers carrying it out; and whilst the aims of
schooling are established by the state and enshrined within league
tables and Ofsted handbooks, teachers are increasingly preoccupied
with the administrative and technical aspects of their work. On the
other hand, the emphasis on such things as flexibility, teamwork, the
construction of mission statements, the formulation of visions and
the preoccupation with semiotic production (Gewirtz *et al.* 1995) are
all characteristics of a post-Taylorist managerialism. Indeed, there
may be good organisational, occupational and service reasons for this
Taylorist/neo-Taylorist 'mix' being almost endemic to public service
organisations. One might suggest that neo-Taylorism embodies the
pressures to rationalise, regulate and generally make more efficient
public service organisations. But it is also clear that public service
organisations have counter tendencies – collegiality, team working,
collaboration, professionalism, quality and trust – that fit poorly
with neo-Taylorism. New managerialism *appears* to address the dimensions of people, values, commitment and purpose that fall outside the
vocabulary of neo-Taylorism (Clarke and Newman 1997).

The commodification and differential valuing of children

Within these new internal regimes of regulation, children have been
recast as commodities. Each 11-year-old child brings to the school a
small pot of money. Each brings the same amount (except if state-
mented) but some students – the ones with a high measured ability
and/or high levels of motivation/parental support – are effectively
worth more than others because they are virtually guaranteed good
examination results with minimal investment. Children with special
educational needs are not valued because they are judged unlikely to
make a valuable contribution to a school's aggregate performance
and are expensive to teach. Working-class children, particularly boys
and more especially white and African-Caribbean working-class

boys, tend to be viewed as potential liabilities in the market place. In contrast, middle-class children, particularly girls and some groups of South Asian children, are prized. It is assumed that these children cost less to teach and that they are more economical in their use of other resources, for example, pastoral care and disciplinary time. In addition, they are seen to contribute favourably to the image of the school. Thus, schools and teachers are effectively encouraged to value students according to what these children can offer the school financially and in terms of exam performance and image. In this way, students have become objects of the education system, to be attracted, excluded, displayed and processed, according to their commercial and semiotic worth, rather than subjects with needs, desires and potentials. They are judged and processed in terms of their perceived capacity to contribute to a school's market success. These judgements not only inform the selection and exclusionary practices of schools, they are also reflected in the new semiologies of schooling (see Gewirtz *et al.* 1995) and they inform the treatment of students within schools. This is evidenced in such things as the growing popularity of a return to traditional internal sorting practices (setting by 'ability'), the devalorisation of special needs and the use of formal pedagogies, which are likely to disadvantage students defined as being of low academic ability.

Hence, the principle of equal value outlined by Daunt (1975), which at least formally structured student-teacher relations in the welfarist era, is being undermined. Of course, in practice, many teachers, probably the majority, did not value children equally under welfarism. Most teachers have probably always favoured, in some respects, those children who are seen as motivated, hard working and likely to perform well in examinations. And the entrenched racism, classism, sexism and heterosexism of school classrooms and systems in the welfarist period has been well documented by researchers. Nonetheless, the structure of funding within the welfarist system was designed to promote the principle of equal value in that the resourcing of schools was governed by calculations of need – however imperfect – rather than roll-size or performance. And in some settings, like London, anti-racist and anti-sexist policies established and maintained a discourse through which issues of worth and equality could be validly articulated. Within such settings, there was space for headteachers and teachers who were genuinely committed to the principle of equal value, to let that principle inform their practice, and to use it to discipline recalcitrant others. It would appear that this kind of space is currently being squeezed out of existence.

A reconfiguration of the social relations of schooling and the subjugation of teachers

Again, it would be romantic and inaccurate to suggest that secondary schools were once democratic, collegial, cooperative institutions, which have been recast in an authoritarian, conflict-ridden mould. However, there was certainly space within the welfarist system for schools to operate in relatively democratic ways in terms of teacher and student participation in the decision-making and day-to-day practices of schools (see, for example, Ball 1987). Furthermore, it is not controversial to argue that teachers in welfarist schools were granted a fair degree of latitude – or a 'licensed autonomy' (Dale 1989) – in curriculum selection and pedagogic approach. Post-welfarism severely limits the scope for participative forms of decision making and autonomous teacher activity. We saw in Chapter 4 how teachers in the case-study schools were having to conform to narrow aims and goals, which are effectively set by the state. Their work was being governed by a technical or instrumental rather than a substantive rationality.

There is a shift not only in vertical relationships but in horizontal ones too. A key technique of managerialism is the creation of internal markets within schools, with departments having to bid against each other for resources and to compete with one another for exam success. 'Teamwork' is encouraged but *within* departmental boundaries, not beyond them. Post-welfarism encourages the pursuit of competitive individualism. Intensification of the labour process of teaching, internal markets, appraisal and the focus on exam performance, all mitigate against the development of cross-disciplinary collaborative enterprises and contribute to a decline in the sociability of school life, as well as to a decline in any authentic sense of common purpose within and between schools. (Although, in some schools, attempts are made to fabricate a common purpose through the promotion of a corporate culture – see Ball 1998.)

It may well also be the case that relations between teachers and students are being reworked as well. I described in Chapter 4 the way in which larger class sizes, the increased proportion of teachers' time taken up by administrative duties and the growing emphasis on results rather than the processes of teaching and learning can work to undermine intimate and complex relationships. These pressures appear to encourage the construction of an instrumental form of 'production line' relations between teachers and students (Bowles and Gintis 1976: 205). Susan Robertson has noted a similar phenomenon in Western Australia:

The intensification of teachers' work inevitably leads to the prioritizing of those activities which are rewarded over those which are not. This is only human. Given that the reward structures for teachers are now based on being able to generate market competitiveness, it is obvious where the sacrifices will be made. However, the more distant teachers become from their students, the more depersonalised their teaching. This leads inexorably to an even further alienated relationship between themselves and their students. Their relationship takes on all the characteristics of the commodity form . . . It is the logic of the market – the commodity form – which has penetrated deep inside schools, and constituted the authority of the new professional.

(Robertson 1996: 45)

The privileging of traditionalist pedagogic regimes

In Chapter 4, I described the ways in which the priorities enshrined in the PWEPC and the practices of new managerialism privileged the adoption of traditional teaching methods in the case-study schools: the return to setting; the increased emphasis on outcomes rather than process; and a more utilitarian, exam-oriented approach to teaching, with less emphasis on responding to the interests of children and the cultivation of positive and rich relationships. These things are accompanied by a pressure and tendency to focus on students on the C–D GCSE borderline and the relative neglect of students who are unlikely to contribute to league-table success (see also Gillborn and Youdell 1999). Larger class sizes are contributing to over-crowded classrooms, which limit opportunities for active learning and encourage a static, didactic blackboard centred approach. In addition, the national curriculum has made life difficult for teachers committed to a non-Anglo-centric curricular content.

Again, I want to reiterate that I am not suggesting that in the welfarist era schools were generally authentically progressive institutions, by which I mean institutions that are run democratically, responsive to the interests and perspectives of students, which encourage active learning and critical thinking and that are attentive to issues of social justice. The majority were not. What I am arguing is that authentically progressive teaching did exist in relatively small pockets of activity but, in the archetypically post-welfarist context where the case-study schools are located, it is being displaced, or at least worn away, by the attritive processes of new managerialism; and the spaces within which authentically progressive practices can be developed have been squeezed.

In addition, it is important to note that those teachers who are still striving to be progressive were trained in higher education (HE) departments of education, which have undergone their own form of post-welfarist transformation. The progressive HE sites within which progressive teachers were once produced would appear to be reinventing themselves in an effort to conform to the traditionalist requirements of Ofsted, the various government circulars which define what trainee teachers should be assessed on, and the Teacher Training Agency's 'national curriculum' for teacher training (Mahony and Hextall 1997). So any new teachers coming through the system keen to adopt progressive pedagogies will find it increasingly difficult to identify – either within their HE institution or school – appropriate role models or sources of inspiration and expertise. They are pressured to adopt traditional pedagogies and so contribute to the reproduction of patterns of division and inequality within schools.

The exacerbation of inequalities of access to schooling and polarisation

All of these developments appear to be contributing towards the reproduction and exacerbation of inequalities and heightened polarisation. These processes can be seen to operate both within individual schools and across school systems.

In effect, oversubscribed schools are displacing responsibility for the more vulnerable children in society to schools that have fewer resources with which to cater for them effectively. The result is differentiated provision and increased social segregation. Working-class children, who are most likely to fail the covert and overt tests of 'ability' and 'motivation' being applied by oversubscribed schools, are on the whole likely to be increasingly ghettoised in undersubscribed, underresourced, understaffed, low-status 'local' schools. Because some racialised groups are disproportionately represented amongst the economically disadvantaged sections of the population, they are more likely to be represented in these 'local' schools; and there is an additional possibility that new methods of selection will prove to be racist. It is also the case that African-Caribbean boys are disproportionately excluded (Bourne *et al.* 1994; Gillborn 1997; SEU 1998). Middle-class white and some South Asian children, on the other hand, are more likely to apply and to be selected for and retained by high-status 'cosmopolitan' schools (Ball *et al*. 1995). This polarisation thesis has been confirmed by a number of studies in a range of national contexts (e.g., Whitty *et al*. 1998; Hughes and Lauder 1999; Noden 2000). At the same time, *within* schools processes of differentiation and segregation are occurring, through setting, and special needs provision is devalued and increased attention is devoted to students most able to contribute to a school's league-table performance (see Chapter 4 in this book; Gewirtz *et al*. 1995; Gillborn and Youdell 1999).

The penetration into schooling of capitalist values and a capitalist mode of rationality

All of the processes described above contribute towards and represent a shift in the mode of rationality and values of schooling – what I referred to in Chapter 3 as values drift. It would appear that post-welfarist schooling operates by means of a capitalist mode of rationality so that what is being valued now in schools are people, practices and forms of relationship which contribute most to commercial success and the maximisation of income. As a result, post-welfarism would appear to have effected a much closer alignment of school values with the values of the capitalist enterprise, with teachers, like workers in the commercial sector, being judged by the quantity of what they produce, their efficiency in producing it and the extent of their loyalty to 'the firm'. Autonomy, creativity, fulfilment and reflexivity are only likely to be valued where they are seen to contribute to productivity. Students, as discussed above, have become commodified and objectified, to be sorted, selected, processed and excluded according to their economic worth. Relationships are instrumental: on the whole, competitive individualism is promoted as the most effective means of maximising productivity; but teamwork is also encouraged when it is likely to enhance quality and productivity. Pedagogical practices are valued and selected in a similarly instrumental fashion, not for the extent to which they might contribute to the development of autonomous, critical, reflective, creative and fulfilled individuals but for the extent to which they might assist in the maximisation of a school's aggregate examination performance. Equity and integration are effectively de-prioritised because commercial success does not (obviously) depend on these things. This is not to argue that schools have totally abandoned any kind of moral or social agenda. In some cases, this is in part because a vigorous moral agenda also makes good marketing sense, as in the case of Martineau School's commitment to feminist goals (Ball and Gewirtz 1997). But many of the teachers I interviewed remained deeply concerned about issues of social justice and integration, which they felt were no longer being addressed. My point is that these commitments sit uneasily alongside the pressure to conform to the demands of the market and are, as a consequence, being marginalised.

The silencing of dissenting voices

In transforming the values and rationality of education provision, post-welfarism seems to have produced a discursive reconstruction of schooling. It would appear that the purposes of schooling have been largely redefined, so that schools are seen primarily as being concerned with the production of measurable short-term learning outcomes. This is both a reflection of and reflected in the rise to prominence of the purveyors of the language and practices of school effectiveness and improvement, with their claims to have developed objective instruments for the identification of failings in schools and the facilitation of improvement. As David Scott (1997) has argued, school effectiveness and improvement is based on a simplistic unilinear model of causation, it often confuses correlation with causation and it rests on a technical-rational model of the relationship between theory and practice:

> Here we refer to a model which understands the practitioner as a technician whose role is to implement objective educational truths, and, therefore, as having a passive role in the implementation process. If it is possible to identify such truths about education, the practitioner who chooses to ignore them is likely to make inadequate judgements about [how] they should proceed in practice.
>
> (Scott 1997: 167)

And, as John White (1997: 52) has pointed out, the emphasis on short-term measurable outcomes, like 'good test scores, GCSE results, low truancy rates or whatever other desiderata the [school effectiveness research] may insist on', means that non-measurable, 'longer-term goals to do with well-roundedness, democratic citizenship, independence of spirit' and so on are neglected. Despite these serious weaknesses, the discourses of school effectiveness and improvement appear to have become hegemonic. And in the new climate of performativity, it would seem that those who question the 'objective educational truths' being 'discovered' by school effectiveness and improvement researchers and who challenge the ideological, pedagogical, social and epistemological assumptions underpinning them are being effectively sidelined in policy terms.

The inculcation of systemic stress

Finally, the compound effect of all of the consequences identified above is the inculcation of systemic stress. Teachers are working longer hours, they are increasingly engaged in tasks which they do not enjoy or value, they are subject to intrusive regimes of inspection, surveillance and judgement, and all within a competitive and increasingly unsociable and under-resourced environment (see Chapter 4). Teachers are increasingly becoming 'bearers' of objective forces (Poulantzas 1973), which they cannot effectively contest. Stress is likely to be most intense in schools located within socio-economically disadvantaged areas where it has been made unfashionable to 'blame' the environment for poor examination results. Teachers, who are struggling to provide on a shoe-string budget an adequate and appropriate education for students who may be hungry, homeless, in care and/or newly arrived in the country, are being stretched to breaking point. But they are now also faced with the fear or reality of redundancy and/or being blamed for 'failing'. As was illustrated in earlier chapters, oversubscribed schools are not immune to stress or inadequate resourcing either. There is always the anxiety, experienced by headteachers and passed on to their staff, that a school's popularity may wane or that a school's budget might be cut because of the local authority's own budgetary problems, and that redundancies may have to be made. In addition, teachers in oversubscribed schools can be faced with the pressure of expanding rolls and larger class sizes within buildings and classrooms not large enough to cater for them. Managers within the case-study schools were very conscious of the existence of stress. It was viewed as something to be managed, a condition to be treated. In this way, stress can be depoliticised, contained and individualised (for example, by teachers being taught techniques to manage stress themselves).

In Part I, I described how the practices of post-welfarism produce stress in teachers but the likelihood is that the stress experienced by teachers will also have consequences for student experiences of schooling. In addition, the traditional pedagogical and sorting practices and the inequality and segregation being promoted by post-welfarism are themselves likely to produce stressed and alienated students.

Having identified the distinguishing features of the lived post-welfarist settlement in education, in concluding this chapter, I want to consider the implications of educational post-welfarism for the problems of the state that post-welfarist policies were meant to help solve.

Post-welfarism, education and the state

I suggested in Chapter 1 that the post-welfarist settlement arose out of three kinds of problem within welfarism – problems of capital accumulation, legitimation and control. The fiscal crisis of the state had created a widely perceived imperative for the reduction of public expenditure in general and education spending in particular. In addition, the perceived decline in the competitiveness of British industry had led attention to be focused on the alleged inadequacy of the state education system in preparing young people with appropriate attitudes and skills for employment. Problems of control, evident in the student 'unrest' of 1968 and the trebling of the strike rate between 1968 and 1972 (CCCS 1981), also focused attention on the perceived inadequacy of schooling, in particular, on the 'loony left-wing' teachers of the metropolises who were supposedly busy fostering the seeds of insurrection rather than conformity in the student population. Finally, the state had faced escalating problems of legitimation. Welfarism had failed in one of its central objectives – to produce greater distributive justice, instead creating a large pool of unemployed and disaffected working-class and young black people. The post-welfarist education settlement sought to resolve these problems by liberating schools from the control of teachers and their unions. It dismantled the institutional infrastructure, attachments and supports of 'social democracy', and attempted a re-acculturation of schooling through markets and devolved management combined with more direct forms of regulation. This was supposed to enable the state to ensure that schooling was more closely aligned both to the requirements of the economy and of social order. Whilst controlling schools and teachers more tightly, the post-welfarist settlement also sought to shift the blame for any failings within the system. The market/management couplet was not only a structural device for regulating schooling but a rhetorical legitimating device that sought to displace responsibility for failing schools from the state to the schools themselves.

In what follows, I want to suggest that each of these problems are potentially exacerbated rather than resolved by post-welfarism. Let me begin with the problem of accumulation. I want to argue that the tighter regime of regulation, which was deemed necessary to produce a closer alignment of schooling to the demands of capital accumulation, may well, in practice, contribute to an intensification of accumulation problems, or at least to a *perception* that accumulation problems are being intensified as a consequence of post-welfarist reforms. The late 1980s and the 1990s saw the emergence of a growing academic and political consensus that Britain's economic success internationally would increasingly be dependent upon it becoming a high-skill, high-wage, high-productivity economy and that education has an important role to play in contributing to such an economy (Finegold and Soskice 1988; CBI 1989; Ashton and Green 1996; Brown and Lauder 1996; DfEE 1997b). This is despite the fact that, as Andy Green (1997: 182) points out, 'Many economists see no proven link between skills and productivity'. But, in a sense, the veracity of the arguments about the relationship between skills and productivity are less significant than the fact that there is a *belief* amongst policy makers that education can contribute to national economic competitiveness. For, in effect, it is *perceptions* of crisis that drive policy; and:

> however valid the economic reasoning, it remains the case that most governments see education and training as the critical factor in national economic performance and competitive advantage.
>
> (Green 1997: 182)

Thus, for example, the Kennedy Report on widening participation in further education (Kennedy 1997a) was based on the premise that:

> Encouraging everyone to participate throughout life in learning, in adding ideas, in increasing their skills and in realizing their full potential is the only way we shall, as a nation, generate new wealth and new jobs. We cannot compete on the basis of cheap labour; we need more people with suitable technical skills, more engaged in research. In short, we need a skilled work force and more educated people in every walk of life.
>
> (Kennedy 1997b: 3)

The post-welfarist educational settlement is increasingly likely to be seen to be working against a high-skills resolution to the perceived crisis of international competitiveness in at least three ways. First, the new managerial regimes of regulation which have been evolving within schools, have produced a stressed and disaffected teaching workforce with increasing numbers leaving the profession.[21] This prompted the Teacher Training Agency to initiate a £1.5 million recruitment campaign in October 1997, but teachers have continued to report a severe, and worsening, crisis of recruitment and retention (STRB 2000c and d). A stressed and depleted teaching workforce is increasingly likely to be viewed as ill-equipped to produce the kinds of highly skilled future workers that are believed to be necessary for Britain to transform itself into a 'high-skill economy'. Second, the polarisation produced by the market/management couplet is also likely to be increasingly viewed as not conducive to the development of a high-skill economy. Ashton and Green (1996) believe, on the basis of their analysis of the newly industrialised economies, that the high-skills route to capital accumulation depends, in part, upon the overwhelming majority of school leavers reaching high levels of achievement in language, science, maths and information technology (IT). The polarisation and exclusion generated by post-welfarism is likely to produce large numbers of students who are leaving school ill-equipped for employment of any kind beyond low-wage, low-skill sweatshop work. Whilst low-skill sweatshop work is unlikely to disappear, even within a so-called high-skill economy, the new consensus seems to be that the majority of workers will need to be highly skilled. Whether or not this is the case, and there is some doubt about whether it is, there is a growing body of opinion which argues that low levels of attainment for large sections of the population in those subject areas deemed to be important – like science, maths and IT – will be damaging for the national economy. There is also a possibility that the return to more traditional methods of teaching, which post-welfarism seems to be producing, will increasingly be viewed as likely to have deleterious economic consequences. One argument that has been put forward is that the 'high-skills route' requires pedagogies that promote active learning, analytical and creative problem-solving skills, particular kinds of initiative and flexibility, rather than the passive imbibing of facts and the ability to regurgitate them in timed examinations, which is what traditional methods are best suited to (Leadbetter 1999; Seltzer and Bentley 1999). The validity of arguments about the link between creativity and employment need to be, and indeed have

---

21 A 1997 survey of 800 secondary and primary schools, commissioned by the *Times Educational Supplement*, found that in secondary schools 37.4 per cent of vacancies were due to ill-health retirement. This compared to 9 per cent of nurses and under 5 per cent of workers in the banking and pharmaceutical industries leaving their posts because of ill-health.

been, questioned (Buckingham 2000). But again, the veracity of these arguments is less relevant here than the fact that their existence may well contribute to the unsettling of the post-welfarist settlement by contributing to a general sense that failings within the schooling system are contributing to a crisis of international competitiveness and accumulation. Hence, the problem of accumulation is essentially also a problem of legitimation.

I want to suggest that there are several other reasons why the market/management device does not seem to be working very effectively as a legitimating mechanism. First, the language of consumer-responsiveness is contradicted by the experiences of many consumers of education. Whilst parents are told they have choice, the experience of many parents is that it is the schools who choose, and that some types of consumer (middle-class ones) are privileged (Gewirtz *et al.* 1995). Second, whilst members of the public may believe the press and the government that the failure of so-called failing schools in working-class areas is the fault of teachers and managers themselves, there are nevertheless high levels of public concern about underinvestment in education by the state. Many middle-class parents who send their children to state schools can see that teachers are trying to do their best in difficult circumstances. In these (non-'failing') schools, difficulties are not viewed to be the responsibility of the school but of the government for not putting enough resources into education and for thereby allowing classes to reach sizes of more than thirty. Such concerns prompted the establishment, in 1994, of FACE (Fights Against Cuts in Education), a mainly middle-class, shire county-based campaigning group, which mobilised parents and teachers to demand more funding for education and reduced class sizes. These were also concerns that New Labour capitalised upon and possibly fuelled in their 1997 election campaign.

Finally, it is doubtful that the restructuring of education can be presented as contributing effectively to solving perceived problems of social control. The idea that schools were responsible for the student and labour unrest in the late 1960s and the 1970s is anyway highly questionable. Very few teachers were probably ever concerned to produce critical and rebellious citizens. But, in any case, if anything, the polarisation and disaffection, which post-welfarist education policies appear to be producing, is more likely to exacerbate rather than solve problems of social control, particularly in urban areas where the effects are most acute. Indeed, it was concerns about the exclusionary effects of post-welfarist policies that contributed to the rise to prominence in the 1990s of ideas around communitarianism and social cohesion (Hughes and Mooney 1998) and which I argue in Chapter 8 account, at least in part, for New Labour's policy emphasis on countering social exclusion through targeted funding and citizenship education.

Conclusions

In this chapter, I began by arguing that it is important not to over-simplify the shift from welfarism to post-welfarism and that there is a need to recognise the diversity of responses to the pressures produced by new organisational and funding arrangements and dominant discourses of performativity and the market. Nevertheless, I have also suggested that there are a number of key trends that can be said to constitute the defining features of post-welfarism and which form the contours within and against which diverse positions are articulated. I went on to argue that these key trends may exacerbate the problems, or perceptions of problems, of capital accumulation, social control and legitimation.

We should not be surprised that the PWEPC has failed to ameliorate the various problems out of which it emerged. After all, as I argued in Chapter 1, it is comprised of a disparate and contradictory set of policies, which emanated from a range of ideological traditions and pragmatic concerns within the Conservative Party that were in tension with each other. What united this diverse range of influences was the common concern to liberate schools from the control of the so-called education establishment, to dismantle the institutional infrastructure and attachments of social democracy and to effect a re-acculturation of schooling. But different fractions of Conservatism were committed to these broad goals for different reasons. Thus, to summarise somewhat crudely: the 'industrial trainers' wanted schools to promote future workers equipped for a modern economy (and even within this fraction there was no consensus about what such preparation ought to involve); neo-liberals wanted schools and teachers to behave in more entrepreneurial, consumer-satisfying ways; and neo-conservatives were concerned about the decline in social order and traditional values. The latter group wanted to '"remoralise" the nation – to root out those causes of decadence which according to Margaret Thatcher and her supporters had contributed so much to Britain's economic and moral decline' (Esland 1996: 26). In addition, there were concerns about the rising cost of welfare in general and education in particular, and a perception of a crisis in public support for the state education system.

To an extent, at least some of these concerns can be interpreted as representing particular formulations of what state theorists identify as the three core problems that drive state policies:

- support of the capital accumulation process
- guaranteeing a context for its continued expansion
- the legitimation of the capitalist mode of production, including the state's own part in it.

(Dale 1989: 28)

As Dale argues, these problems:

> are writ small in the education system. [The state] may be required to find solutions in all three core problem areas simultaneously and it is unable to do so. In education, as elsewhere, these solutions are often mutually contradictory.

(Dale 1989: 31)

But the policies were not just a response to these problems. As Dale has pointed out, 'the core problems do not account for everything either the State or the education system does' (1989: 30). Thus, for example, the neo-conservative preoccupation with the restoration of respect for the family, property and authority cannot be reduced to a concern about guaranteeing a context for the continued expansion of capital accumulation. Similarly, the neo-liberal desire to make the education system function in more consumer-satisfying ways, although in large part rooted in concerns about economic efficiency and to some extent prompted by concerns about the need to restore social order and public faith in the education system, was also grounded in arguments about the ethical desirability of choice and autonomy.

That the educational reforms of successive Conservative governments failed to resolve the tensions between the various ideological, economic and political agendas out of which they emerged is also a point made by Geoff Esland (1996). Writing about post-compulsory education, towards the end of the 17 year period of Conservative rule, Esland argued that:

> The contradictions which arise for the British Conservative state from trying to legitimate the different underlying rationales of its education and training policies have become increasingly transparent. Any pretence at universalism is challenged by its preference for selective education and 'opting out'; the notion of parental and

student 'choice' is countered by the tendency for 'successful' institutions themselves to select their student intake; the rhetoric of commitment to raising 'standards' and 'quality' is met by the reality of underfunding . . . arguments for highly skilled workers in a 'knowledge-based' society are undermined by a deregulated labour market and the lack of an industrial policy which could help to generate such jobs; and the provision of an 'education for the twenty-first century' has to overcome both the conceptually deficient, competence-based system of vocational education and training and the prevailing emphasis on cultural nationalism within the school curriculum.

(Esland 1996: 65)

A further contradiction that lies at the heart of the post-welfarist reforms is a tension – probably irreconcilable – around the treatment of teachers, in particular around how much autonomy they should be given. The problem for the state in this respect is how to achieve a workable balance between licence and regulation (Dale 1989). The advantage of licensed autonomy is that it has the potential to produce a motivated and committed workforce able to invest energy and creativity into the educational process. However, too much licence means that what is taught may not always satisfy the perceived requirements of the state and the economy. Regulated autonomy, on the other hand, enables tighter control of what is taught and how it is done but, as the research reported in Part I has demonstrated, it also fosters stress and hostility, which is deleterious to the production of an education system appropriately sensitive and responsive to the perceived demands of the state and the economy. In other words, it would appear that a central dilemma for policy makers in education is that when teachers are awarded too much licence they *do not* necessarily do what is required of them; but if their work is over-regulated they *cannot* do what is required of them. As Jenny Ozga (2000) argues, neither management strategy is stable. Direct regulation has historically been associated with teacher militancy and system inefficiency, whilst licence, in the form 'of an ideology of professionalism creates the potential for teachers to extend the terms of their licence to an unacceptable degree, as they did in the 1970s in England' (Ozga 2000).

In the final chapter of this book, I will consider the extent to which New Labour's 'third way' for education is likely to resolve the major tensions identified in this chapter. But, before doing that, in Chapter 7 I want to explore, more explicitly than has been possible in this chapter, the social justice implications of educational post-welfarism.

7 Post-welfarist schooling

A social justice audit

A central feature of the post-welfarist reforms in education and other welfare sectors has been what Michael Power (1997) has referred to as the audit explosion, which he describes in the following way:

> During the late 1980s and early 1990s, the word 'audit' began to be used . . . with growing frequency in a wide variety of contexts. In addition to the regulation of private company accounting by financial audit, practices of environmental audit, value for money audit, management audit, forensic audit, data audit, intellectual property audit, medical audit, teaching audit, and technology audit emerged, and, to varying degrees, acquired a degree of institutional stability and acceptance. Increasing numbers of individuals and organizations found themselves subject to new or more intensive accounting and audit requirements. In short, a growing population of 'auditees' began to experience a wave of formalized and detailed checking up on what they do.
>
> (Power 1997: 3)

The audit explosion is clearly manifest in schools, which, as a consequence of the 1992 Education (Schools) Act, have to undergo regular Ofsted inspections. In addition, it is now commonplace for pre-Ofsted 'mock' inspections to be carried out by local authorities to help headteachers and teachers prepare for the 'real thing'. Moreover, if Ofsted detect failings, schools may be re-inspected by the local authority to check up on how they are progressing in relation to their post-Ofsted 'action plan' before being subjected to a further re-inspection by Ofsted.

Inspections of schools are framed by a whole range of criteria. They include: students' academic attainment and progress; their attitudes, behaviour and personal development; their spiritual, moral, social and cultural development; attendance; the quality of teaching, curriculum, assessment, support and guidance; and the management and efficiency of schools. Whilst these are not necessarily incompatible with social justice, there was – until the revision of the inspection framework in January 2000 following the publication of the Macpherson Report (see Chapter 8) – little explicit expectation within Ofsted's documentation that schools would attend to social justice issues. Consequently, schools could perform well in Ofsted inspections, without necessarily having devoted any attention to the promotion of social justice. Indeed, one of the effects of the audit explosion and associated reforms in education under successive Conservative governments was the active marginalisation of concerns about social justice. In the process of making themselves auditable, schools were under pressure to emphasise and make visible those things they were being checked up on and, in the process of emphasising these things, various forms of oppression were produced.

The aim of this chapter is to map out, and conduct, on the basis of insights derived from earlier chapters in the book, a different kind of audit. First, I want to make some suggestions about what shape a framework for carrying out a social justice audit in education might take and then I will apply it to post-welfarist schooling as it has emerged in the 1980s and 1990s.

Developing a framework for a social justice audit: Young's 'five faces of oppression'

Given the centrality of issues of social justice to so much policy-sociology research in education, surprisingly little attention has been devoted to exploring precisely what we mean, or ought to mean, when we talk about social justice. Yet, if we want to understand the extent and ways in which policies contribute to, or detract from, the promotion of social justice in education, then we need to be clear about what definition of social justice we are using.

In her seminal text, *Justice and the Politics of Difference*, Young (1990) argues for an extension of the boundaries of what is usually thought of as social justice. She suggests that social justice should not be used exclusively in the narrow conventional sense of referring to the way in which goods are distributed in society. Rather, Young thinks it should be expanded to include 'all aspects of institutional rules and relations insofar as they are subject to potential collective action' (Young 1990: 16). Following Young, I want to suggest that it is useful to think of social justice as comprising two broad dimensions – one distributional, the other relational.

The *distributional* dimension refers to the principles by which goods are distributed in society. This is the conventional conception of social justice, classically defined by Rawls as follows:

> The subject matter of justice is the basic structure of society, or more exactly, the way in which the major social institutions . . . distribute fundamental rights and duties and determine the distribution of advantages from social cooperation.
>
> (Rawls 1972: 7)

For Rawls, the concept of justice refers to 'a proper balance between competing claims'. How goods are distributed is clearly a vital component of how we treat each other. However, to 'read' social justice as being *exclusively* about distribution is severely limiting and it is important that we conceptualise social justice in a broader way.

The *relational* dimension refers to the nature of the relationships that structure society. A focus on this second dimension helps us to theorise about issues of power and how we treat each other, both in the sense of micro-level face-to-face interactions and in the sense of macro social and economic relations, which are mediated by institutions like the state and the market. For Rawls, justice is about the distribution of rights, duties and the social and economic goods accruing from social cooperation. It does not appear to be concerned with the *form* of social cooperation itself. It is the form of social cooperation – i.e., the political/relational system within which the distribution of social and economic goods, rights and responsibilities takes place – which is the concern of the relational dimension. In one sense, this can be conceived of as another dimension of distributive justice in that in part it refers to the way in which relations of power are distributed in society. But relational justice is not just concerned with the *distribution* of power relations. Nor is it just concerned with the *procedures* by which goods are distributed in society (commonly referred to as *procedural* justice). Relational justice might *include* procedural justice but it denotes more than this. It is about the *nature* and *ordering* of social relations, the formal and informal rules that govern how members of society treat each other both on a macro level and at a micro-interpersonal level. Thus, it refers to the practices and procedures that govern the organisation of political systems, economic and social institutions, families and one-to-one social relationships. These things cannot unproblematically be conceptually reduced to matters of distribution.

One way of distinguishing between the distributional and relational dimensions is by thinking of them as rooted within two contrasting ontological perspectives. The distributional dimension is essentially individualistic and atomistic, in that it refers to how goods are distributed to individuals in society. In Miller's formulation, it means 'ensuring everyone receives their due' (Miller 1976: 20). By contrast, the relational dimension is holistic and non-atomistic, being essentially concerned with the nature of inter-connections between individuals in society, rather than with how much individuals get.

It could be argued that in separating out social justice into these two dimensions I am creating a false distinction. Such an argument would go something along these lines:

> Social justice is about the distribution of goods. Whilst goods are more usually narrowly conceived as referring to material things, the definition of goods can and has been extended, as it was by Rawls, to include non-tangible things, for example, particular forms of relationships. If relationships are goods, then the distinction disintegrates.

Whilst this argument might be logical, I would nevertheless argue that it is extremely worthwhile thinking about the two dimensions as separate, albeit strongly connected. If we were to prioritise matters of distribution and treat relationships as merely goods to be distributed, then we may neglect proper consideration of the nature of those relational goods to be distributed. As Young has argued, the 'logic of redistribution' leads us to focus upon 'what individual persons have, how much they have, and how that amount compares to what other persons have' rather than on 'what people are doing, according to what institutionalized rules, how their doings and havings are structured by institutionalized relations that constitute their positions, and how the combined effect of their doings has recursive effects on their lives' (Young, 1990: 25). Concepts like power, opportunity and self-respect are misrepresented, if subsumed into the distributional paradigm, because they are more about 'doing' than 'having'. To illustrate this point, Young takes the example of opportunities. Within the distributional paradigm, opportunities are made to sound like discrete goods that we can be allocated more or less of. In contrast, Young argues that 'opportunity is a concept of enablement rather than possession' (1990: 26). As a result, it is wrong to think of opportunities as things which are *distributed.* We have opportunities if we are not constrained from doing things or if the conditions within which we live enable us to do them. Therefore, the extent to which we have opportunities depends upon the enabling possibilities generated by the rules and practices of the society within which we operate, and by the ways in which people treat each other in that society. So making a judgement about the extent of opportunities we have involves 'evaluating not a distributive outcome but the social structures that enable or constrain the individuals in relevant situations' (1990: 26). In short, by isolating relational justice as a separate dimension, we are forced to think in greater depth about the nature of the relationships that structure society and that structure what we do, what we have and the effects of what we do and have on our lives.

Young's particular approach to relational justice rests on a conceptualisation of *injustice* based on a detailed explication of five 'faces' of oppression: exploitation, marginalisation, powerlessness, cultural imperialism and violence. Young argues that: 'Distributive injustices may contribute to and result from these forms of oppression, but none is reducible to distribution and all involve social structures and relations beyond distribution' (Young 1990: 9). Young's framework provides us with a wide-ranging set of questions, which can be used to inform evaluations of education policies from a social justice perspective. More specifically, as I have argued elsewhere (Gewirtz 1998), they lead us to ask how, to what extent and why education policies support, interrupt or subvert:

1   exploitative relationships (capitalist, patriarchal, racist, heterosexist, disablist, etc.) within and beyond schools
2   processes of marginalisation and inclusion within and beyond the school system
3   the promotion of relationships based on recognition, respect, care and mutuality, or the production of powerlessness (for education workers and students)
4   practices of cultural imperialism within and beyond schools, and
5   violent practices within and beyond the school system.

The strength of Young's approach lies in the way it builds upon and draws together insights from Marxist, feminist, anti-racist and postmodernist approaches to justice. Marxists challenged Rawls on the grounds that he took for granted and obscured the unequal and exploitative class relations that form the context of Rawls' theory of justice (Macpherson 1973; Nielson 1978). Young suggests that this

Marxist critique provides a useful basis upon which to develop a relational conception of justice because it brings into view the institutional context within which distributions occur. But Young also draws on feminist, anti-racist and post-modernist critiques of Marxism's narrow focus on class as the only axis of social difference that is seen to matter. In addition, Young takes seriously post-modernist concerns about Marxism's exclusive concern with structure, specifically capitalism, and its consequent neglect of micro-level face-to-face interactions. Thus, for Young, institutional context is understood in a broader sense than 'mode of production':

> It includes any structures or practices, the rules and norms that guide them, and the language and symbols that mediate social interactions within them, in institutions of state, family, and civil society, as well as the workplace. These are relevant to judgements of justice and injustice insofar as they condition people's ability to participate in determining their actions and their ability to develop and exercise their capacities.
>
> (Young 1990: 22)

This broad definition of institutional context enables a focus on the way in which structures, practices, rules, norms, languages and symbols of all kinds – not just capitalist ones – operate. And it prompts us to explore how some structures and practices can produce (and, in turn, may be produced by) face-to-face social interactions characterised by a lack of mutual recognition and respect that are based upon classist, racist, sexist, heterosexist, ageist or disablist assumptions.

In what follows, I want to draw upon Young's expanded conceptualisation of social justice to explore how and to what extent the structures, practices, language and social relations of post-welfarist schooling promote or inhibit the ability of teachers and students to, first, develop and exercise their capacities, and second, do so within conditions that they have participated in determining. In order to do this, I will focus specifically on the impact of the policies of successive Conservative administrations in the 1980s and 1990s.

The audit

I have argued that social justice is most usefully understood in a broad sense to encompass two dimensions – the distributional and the relational. If, for the moment, we conceive of justice in its purely distributional sense, it would appear from the available evidence that post-welfarist policies exacerbate injustice through the promotion of inequalities of access to schooling and of polarisation in their composition. As I argued in Chapter 6, a range of studies in different national contexts suggest that, where markets operate, working-class and minority ethnic children are increasingly concentrated in under-resourced schools whilst middle-class children are more likely to attend relatively well-resourced schools (Whitty *et al.* 1998; Hughes and Lauder 1999; Noden 2000). This effectively means that educational resources are being redistributed from the least to the most advantaged sections of society. Within schools similar processes of resource redistribution have occurred through such processes as the devalorisation of special needs provision, setting and the emphasis on providing for 'able' or 'gifted' children.

But in what ways is post-welfarism contributing to the exacerbation of relational injustice? I now want to apply Young's criteria, in order to explore the extent and ways in which teachers and students may be oppressed by post-welfarist policies, processes and practices. In doing so, I will explicate each 'face' of oppression a little more extensively than I did in the previous section.

Exploitation

Both the concept of exploitation and whether or not teachers represent an exploited group have long been topics of considerable debate amongst Marxist scholars (Roemer 1982; Wright 1985, 1988; Lawn and Ozga 1988; Watkins 1992). There is not space here to enter into these debates but I want to capture some key elements, in order to draw attention to the usefulness of Young's conceptualisation of exploitation. Marx defined exploitation in a technical economic sense to describe the relationship between bourgeoisie and proletariat. On this definition, exploitation is a social process by which the 'surplus product of the direct producers (that is, the product over and above what they require in specific historical circumstances, for their continued labouring existence) is appropriated by the dominant, owning class' (Zeitlin 1980: 2). The viability of the theory of surplus value upon which Marx's theory of exploitation is based has been called into question by those who argue that it cannot accommodate the increasing complexity of capitalist economies, in which many workers are engaged in the production of 'invisible commodities' (Hunt 1977; Lawn and Ozga 1988). Marx's theory of exploitation has also been criticised for being too narrow to accommodate or adequately explain gender or racial exploitation (Giddens 1981; Bowles and Gintis 1986).

It is in response to such problems, that Young broadens the concept of exploitation. Drawing upon Macpherson's (1973) reconstruction of Marx's theory of exploitation and other insights from the debates summarised above, Young defines exploitation as a form of oppression, which 'occurs through a steady process of the transfer of the results of the labor of one social group to benefit another' (Young 1990: 49). She is careful to distinguish exploitation from the broader category of domination. For Young, domination 'consists in persons having to perform actions whose rules and goals they have not participated in determining, under institutionalized conditions they have not had a part in deciding' (Young 1990: 218). Domination only becomes exploitation when the actions someone has to perform, under conditions they have not participated in deciding, *systematically benefit another without reciprocation* (Young 1990: 218). Hence, for Young:

> The injustice of capitalist society consists in the fact that some people exercise their capacities under the control, according to the purposes, and for the benefit of other people. Through the private ownership of the means of production, and through markets that allocate labor and the ability to buy goods, capitalism systematically transfers the powers of some persons to others, thereby augmenting the power of the latter. In this process of the transfer of powers . . . the capitalist class acquires and maintains an ability to extract benefit from workers. Not only are powers transferred from workers to capitalists, but also the powers of workers diminish by more than the amount of transfer, because workers suffer material deprivation and a loss of control, and hence are deprived of important elements of self respect.
>
> (Young 1990: 49)

One of the attractions of Young's conceptualisation of exploitation is that it addresses crucial shortcomings of Marx's theory by drawing attention to the specificities of different forms of exploitation. Thus, for Young, exploitation can occur in the restricted Marxist sense of appropriating surplus value. But, by defining exploitation as the transfer of energies from one group to another, Young is also able to identify two aspects to gender exploitation: 'transfer of fruits of material labor to men and transfer of nurturing and sexual energies to men' (Young 1990: 50).

Young's conceptualisation of exploitation can help us map out the complex web of exploitative relations that exist in and around schools. First, it can help us see how teachers are both exploiters of others and how they represent an exploited group themselves. For example, on Young's definition, teachers, as professionals, are exploiters of non-professionals, in that the 'material' work of non-professionals – like cleaning classrooms, cooking dinners, typing letters – frees teachers for the 'higher' work of 'thinking, designing and calculating . . . making decisions, writing reports, planning, and coordinating and supervizing' (Young 1990: 218–19). However, since the 1970s, a number of commentators, in the UK, North America and elsewhere, have observed that, in many ways, teachers' work is becoming deskilled, with the diminution of the thinking, designing and calculating parts of the job, as teachers are increasingly expected to execute decisions made elsewhere (Ozga 1988). But, even in such circumstances, the relationship between teachers and non-professionals in schools is nevertheless, on Young's definition, exploitative:

> because the professionals usually get paid more, get more recognition, and have greater power and authority, even though the work of some nonprofessionals directly enables their work.
>
> (Young 1990: 219)

On the other hand, teachers themselves can be viewed as exploited in a number of senses. For example, it can be argued that teachers are exploited by those who manage them, in that teachers' increasingly technicist work frees school managers for yet 'higher' work; and the higher pay, power and authority that managers accrue is directly enabled by the work of teachers. Exploitation in schools, as in most other workplaces, is gendered and racialised to the extent that women and minority ethnic groups tend to predominate in jobs with the lowest pay and status – for example, as classroom assistants and mealtime supervisors – whilst the highest paying high-status jobs tend to be held by white men. It can also be argued that teachers *and managers* in schools are exploited (if less directly) by private employers, in that the energy teachers and headteachers expend in 'producing' educated workers might enable employers to extract value from those workers, the benefits of which are not transferred back to workers in schools. Furthermore, it is possible to argue that teachers and managers in schools are exploited by those professional and managerial workers in the private and public sectors who are more highly paid and have more status and authority than those who work in schools. This relationship can be classified as exploitative where the higher pay, status and authority of such professional/managerial groups depends on the existence of the educated labour 'produced' by workers in schools.

The extent and ways in which the web of exploitative relationships in and around schools has been, or is in the process of being, *transformed*, as a consequence of post-welfarist policies, is a complex issue. Certainly, it is difficult to see how post-welfarist policies, have done anything to interrupt processes of exploitation within and around schools, and it is possible to construct an argument that the exploitation of teachers has been intensified, along the lines that they have had to be more productive to serve other people's needs whilst deriving less personal fulfilment from their work.

First of all, teachers have lost out materially as a consequence of post-welfarist policies. In Chapter 4, I pointed out that a number of surveys support the perceptions of teachers I interviewed that they were working longer hours in the 1990s than they were in the 1970s (NAS/UWT 1990 and 1991; ILO 1991; Lowe 1991; Campbell and St J. Neill 1994; STRB 1996, 2000a and 2000b). At the same time, there has been a long-term decline in teachers' salaries since the fiscal crisis of the mid-1970s (which arguably marked the beginning of the decline of welfarism) in relation to the average increase in earnings of non-manual workers. I have also pointed to evidence that suggests that opportunities for participative forms of decision making and autonomous teacher activity have probably become more tightly circumscribed now that teachers' work is scrutinised more intensively by external agencies and governed increasingly by a technical, rather than substantive, rationality. In Chapter 6, I suggested that the compound effect of all of these factors – the additional workload, the decline in participative decision making and autonomy, as well as increased surveillance and the deteriorating quality of relationships in schools - is the inculcation of stress.

It could thus be argued that, as teachers have increasingly been deprived both in material terms and in terms of control and personal fulfilment, and as their working hours have increased, they have experienced intensified exploitation by all of those (employers and professional/managerial workers in both the private and public sectors) whose material and status well-being is dependent on the extraction of value from educated labour. It is also possible to construct an argument along similar lines that managers in schools have experienced intensified exploitation.

The picture is, however, complicated by the fact that teachers do not constitute a homogenous social group but represent a group cross-cut by gender, ethnicity, class background, disability, age and so on. More work needs to be done in mapping the changing degrees, experiences and modes of exploitation of different fractions within the teaching workforce.

And what of students? To what extent and in what ways can it be argued that they represent an exploited group, and what has been the impact of post-welfarism on the nature of their exploitation? On Young's definition of exploitation as the transfer of energies from one group to another, it is possible to argue that students have always been an exploited group. For the way in which students exercise their capacities in the vast majority of schools has never been determined solely by a conception of children's own needs and interests. Rather children's energies are used to augment the interests of others to the extent that what students do in schools is shaped by a perception of what is in the interests of schools, parents, employers and the state.

However, these more instrumental purposes of schooling have arguably become more dominant in the post-welfarist reconstruction of education. Part I highlighted the more overt commodification of students and the increased adoption of narrow, instrumentalist and didactic pedagogic practices that the post-welfarist education policy complex has contributed to producing (see also Gewirtz *et al.* 1995; Woods *et al.* 1997; Smyth and Shacklock 1998; Woods and Jeffrey 1998). And in Chapter 6 I argued that this commodification represents a much closer alignment of school values with the values of the capitalist enterprise, where the focus is on what students can offer the school, rather than on what the school can offer them.

But, like teachers, students are a heterogeneous group. There is, therefore, considerable work to be done in exploring the multiple forms of exploitation that post-welfarist policies produce or interrupt, and there is a need to focus on the differentiated ways in which exploitation is, or is not, experienced by students of different 'abilities', classes, genders, and racialised groupings.

Marginalisation

Young defines marginalisation as a form of oppression in which people are 'expelled from useful participation in social life and thus potentially subjected to severe material deprivation and even extermination' (1990: 53). But:

> Marginalization does not cease to be oppressive when one has shelter and food . . . Even if marginals were provided a comfortable material life within institutions that respected their freedom and

dignity, injustices of marginality would remain in the form of use-lessness, boredom, and lack of self-respect. Most of our society's productive and recognized activities take place in contexts of organized social cooperation, and social structures and processes that close persons out of participation in such social cooperation are unjust. Thus while marginalization definitely entails serious issues of distributive justice, it also involves the deprivation of cultural, practical and institutionalized conditions for exercising capacities in a context of recognition and interaction.

(Young 1990: 55)

The practices of post-welfarism marginalise particular categories of children first by devaluing them. In earlier chapters I have drawn attention to the way certain categories of children, for example, those classified as having special needs and African-Caribbean and white working-class boys, tend not to be valued within a post-welfarist policy environment because they are judged to be particularly demanding on resources and/or unlikely to be able to make a significant positive contribution to a school's examinations league-table performance. Students classified as belonging to those categories tend not to be selected for, and are more likely to be excluded from, the schools that are the most generously resourced and considered to be the most socially desirable. Hence, it would seem that the most vulnerable students are marginalised within post-welfarist contexts by being ghettoised within institutions that lack the resources to adequately serve their needs. *Inside* schools, the same groups of students are also marginalised by the increased adoption of setting practices. If we are to extrapolate from existing research on the effects of the grouping of students by 'ability' (e.g., Oakes 1990; Slavin 1996; Hallam and Toutounji 1996; Boaler 1997a; Sukhnandan and Lee 1998) then it is reasonable to conclude that the combination of these processes of selection, exclusion *and* setting is likely to have intensified significantly, amongst marginalised students, the experiences of boredom and perceptions of uselessness identified by Young as key consequences of marginalisation. Thus, there are cultural as well as distributional injustices associated with the marginalisation of students.

As far as teachers are concerned, those who are still in work have not been marginalised in the sense of being excluded from 'useful participation in social life', although many teachers may have *felt* marginalised by some of the processes and practices of post-welfarism, as a consequence of their experiences of exploitation. Moreover, learning and language support teachers, who are especially involved in dealing with those students who are most marginalised by post-welfarism, may well have experienced a form of *reflected marginalisation*. Special needs teachers have certainly been particularly vulnerable to the new 'flexible' staffing practices and to redundancy (Gewirtz *et al.* 1995).

Powerlessness

Just as teachers may have felt marginalised by their experiences of exploitation, so many may, justifiably, also have felt that they lack power, which Young defines as the ability of people to participate in decisions that affect the conditions of their lives. I have argued that, in effect, it would seem that managerial modes of coordination produce subjugated classroom teachers, teachers who have lost control of what they teach, how they teach and the determination of the goals of their teaching, and who have to live in the shadow of constant surveillance. Whilst some researchers have detected a heightened sense of profes-sionalism amongst *primary* teachers (e.g., Campbell and St J. Neill 1994b), enhanced professionalism was not a prominent feature of the perceptions of teachers in the secondary schools I have studied and nor were the 'new' professionalism and collaborative teaching cultures that Hargreaves (1994) describes. The experiences of teachers I inter-viewed came closer to those who participated in Robertson and Soucek's (1991) study of teachers in Western Australia:

> In essence, the changes have meant teachers can participate in making decisions over a limited range of technical issues, not the big ticket items such as: What is it that we want children to know? How do we provide opportunities for students to genuinely participate in the learning process? What does it mean to educate a critical citizenry? Instead teachers have been left to dream up schemes as to how they can work smarter to increase student per-formance, compete for scarce students with neighbouring schools, raise money from the business sector, or access new technology for the school through school-business partnerships. At the same time it has marginalized teachers' dissenting voices and reduced their scope for critical practice and autonomy.
> (Robertson 1996: 43–4; see also Woods *et al.* 1997)

However, whilst they may have suffered a loss of power under post-welfarism in relation to school managers and the state, teachers are not powerless, nor have they been rendered powerless by post-welfarism. As Young has argued, in advanced capitalist countries:

most workplaces are not organized democratically, direct participation in public policy decisions is rare, and policy implementation
is for the most part hierarchical, imposing rules on bureaucrats
and citizens. Thus most people in these societies do not regularly
participate in making decisions that affect the conditions of their
lives and actions, and in this sense most people lack significant
power.

(Young 1990: 56)

But, drawing on a Foucauldian conception of power, Young also
points out that:

domination in modern society is enacted through the widely dis-
persed powers of many agents mediating the decisions of others.
To that extent many people have some power in relation to
others, even though they lack the power to decide policies or
results. The powerless are those who lack authority or power
even in this mediated sense, those over whom power is exercised
without their exercising it; the powerless are situated so that they
must take orders and rarely have the right to give them.

(Young 1990: 56)

In the context of post-welfarist schools, teachers may have experienced
a loss of power, to the extent that they may have felt – and indeed been
– less involved in school decision making but they have continued to
exercise power on a daily basis over students, and some teachers
have continued to exercise power over other teachers. Most students
are more appropriately defined as powerless within schools, since
they regularly have power exercised over them but rarely have the
opportunity to exercise power over others (although, of course, some
do exercise power over other students by various forms of bullying
and harassment). However, whilst it is difficult to construct a *conclusive*
case for arguing that the powerlessness of students has been intensified,
a clear sign of increased powerlessness is the reduced evidence of the
social agency of students in the form of rebellion or riot in the 1990s
compared to the 1970s and 1980s.

Cultural imperialism

According to Young:

To experience cultural imperialism means to experience how the dominant meanings of society render the particular perspective of one's own group invisible at the same time as they stereotype one's group and mark it out as the Other.

Cultural imperialism involves the universalization of a dominant group's experience and culture, and its establishment as the norm.

(Young 1990: 58–9)

The instrumentalism, narrowness of focus and pedagogic tradition-alism of post-welfarist schooling under Conservative governments may be viewed as having functioned as mechanisms of cultural imperi-alism in two senses. First, as I argued in Chapter 6, these mechanisms appear to have functioned in such a way as to marginalise dissenting voices and to squeeze the spaces within which emancipatory practices, which promote, what Young calls, self development, can evolve. Second, the mechanisms of pedagogic traditionalism and narrowness of focus associated with the discourse of performativity themselves have represented new possibilities for the promotion of culturally imperialist practices in schools, including an ethno-centric curriculum and ethno-centric pedagogies.

However, it is important to remember that cultural imperialism has a long history in English schools. This was highlighted particularly by the 'new' sociologists of education in the 1970s, who argued that the way schools were organised and their curricula and pedagogies reflected the experiences, values, interests and ways of learning of dominant (i.e., middle-class) social groups (Young 1971). This form of critique was extended by feminist and anti-racist teachers in the 1980s, and gave rise to the advocacy and adoption in some schools of feminist and anti-racist policies and practices (Coard 1971; ALTARF 1979; Deem 1980; Arnot and Weiner 1987). As I have emphasised in previous chapters, I do not wish to imply that prior to the introduction of post-welfarist policies *most* schools or teachers were especially attentive to issues of social justice. Nor do I want to give the impression that their introduction marked an end to teachers struggling within their own classrooms to develop practices rooted in a recognition of, and a respect for, difference. There were – and still are – teachers who, *in spite of* the pressures towards ethno-centrism generated by post-welfarist policies, are able to develop curricula designed to engage a diversity of students with the kinds of critical political, moral and social issues associated with a politics of recognition (Fraser 1997) that are not covered in the national curriculum (as in the case of Ruskin's head of humanities cited in Chapter 4 – see also Hill and Cole 1999). However, what I am suggesting is that in the welfarist era there were more spaces for teachers who wanted to develop within schools organisational practices, curricula and pedagogies, which were underpinned by a recognition and respect for diverse cultural identities and by a desire to combat culturally imperialist school practices.

Violence

Young includes in the category of violence not only physical attacks but 'harassment, intimidation or ridicule simply for the purpose of degrading, humiliating, or stigmatising group members' (Young 1990: 61). For Young:

> What makes violence a phenomenon of social injustice and not merely an individual wrong, is its existence as a social practice.
>
> Violence is systematic because it is directed at members of a group simply because they are members of that group . . . The oppression of violence consists not only in direct victimization, but in the daily knowledge shared by all members of oppressed groups that they are liable to violation, solely on account of their group identity. Just living under such a threat of attack on oneself or family or friends deprives the oppressed of freedom and dignity, and needlessly expends their energy . . .
>
> To the degree that institutions and social practices encourage, tolerate, or enable the perpetration of violence against members of specific groups, those institutions and practices are unjust and should be reformed.
>
> (Young 1990: 62–3)

Violence, in the form of physical attacks as well as harassment, of a racist, sexist and disablist nature, has continued to occur in schools in the post-welfarist era, as it did under welfarism. It certainly could not be argued that in general post-welfarist schools have encouraged or tolerated the perpetration of violence against members of specific groups. There are grounds for concern, however, that, through the mechanisms of cultural imperialism discussed above, post-welfarist policies may have prevented schools from doing as much as they should to challenge the kinds of attitudes that underpin group-directed violence. There is, therefore, an urgent need to interrogate post-welfarist policies from this perspective.

Conclusion

The preceding analysis strongly suggests that the post-welfarist policies of successive Conservative administrations in the 1980s and 1990s have exacerbated educational injustices, both distributional and relational, in various ways. In particular, it would seem that: educational resources have effectively been redistributed away from the most vulnerable and towards the most privileged groups of children in society; exploitation of teachers has been intensified; working-class students, particularly boys, and some racialised groups of students have been increasingly marginalised; and opportunities to develop 'pedagogies of recognition' and to undermine the culturally imperialist practices of schools have been heavily circumscribed.

However, 1997 saw the election of a New Labour government, which was re-elected in 2001. New Labour are formally committed to social justice and to combating social exclusion. Particularly in the wake of Sir William Macpherson's report (Macpherson 1999) on the police investigation into the murder of the black teenager, Stephen Lawrence, New Labour appeared to place a renewed emphasis on the need to combat racism and to promote the values of citizenship in schools. On paper, at least, such proclamations suggested that some of the currents of Conservative post-welfarism may have become a thing of the past. In the following chapter, I look more closely at New Labour's educational agenda and ask whether, in fact, such optimism is justified.

8 Towards a new educational settlement?

New Labour's 'third way' for education

During its first term in office, New Labour introduced fresh legislation at a frenetic pace. Alongside their education reforms, new organisational arrangements were put in place for local government, health, social services, housing, and the criminal justice and benefits systems. The government went to some lengths to present their policies as distinct from those of their Conservative predecessors, drawing in particular on the rhetorical device of the 'third way'. Clarke and Newman's analysis of New Labour policy texts reveals how the 'third way' operates as a 'discursive practice' whose 'practical function is to define the impossibility of alternatives' (1998: 6). New Labour texts thereby tell a story of:

> past failures in order to create space for the 'third way'. The failures of statism are juxtaposed against the failures of the internal market or unregulated grass roots activity as the conditions which both necessitate and legitimate a new approach . . . The 'third way' is produced as the only viable or reasonable option.
>
> (Clarke and Newman 1998: 7–8)

The third way, as a rhetorical figure, clearly has an important role to play in the legitimation of New Labour policies. However, it is with the third way as a *political programme* that this chapter is concerned. More specifically, the chapter considers the key components of New Labour's agenda for education and asks: to what extent do third way policies in education represent a continuation of, or a departure from, the policies of successive Conservative governments in the 1980s and 1990s? What will be the consequences of third way policies for social justice? How successful are these policies likely to be in resolving the tensions generated by the post-welfarist settlement? And to what extent can

New Labour's third way be said to constitute the beginnings of a new educational settlement?

The third way in education

The apparently contradictory nature of New Labour's political project has prompted Geoff Andrews (1999) to coin for it the paradoxical label 'neo-liberal humanism'. Certainly, New Labour's education policies appear to combine elements of the neo-liberalism that was characteristic of New Right policies with humanistic elements more commonly associated with a social democratic stance. However, Andrews' designation fails to capture the moral authoritarian components of New Labour's policy mix, which are particularly apparent in the fields of education, family policy and criminal justice, and which to some extent draw upon the neo-conservative strand of New Right thinking. New Labour's third way might, therefore, be more accurately described as constituting a neo-liberal authoritarian humanism. In this section I want to begin by outlining the neo-liberal and authoritarian elements of New Labour's third way for education before going on to identify its apparently more humanistic components. In subsequent sections I will examine the tensions within and likely consequences of this complex amalgam of policy strategies.

The neo-liberal and authoritarian elements of New Labour's third way are largely couched in the language of 'quality' and, like their Conservative predecessors, New Labour has drawn on a range of 'quality' strategies borrowed from the private sector. In the private sector there is, as Kirkpatrick and Martinez-Lucio point out, 'no clear unified programme of quality improvement, but a wide variety of approaches which have in common only the most basic objective of somehow increasing the competitive advantage and profitability of a firm' (1995: 7). But, broadly speaking, private-sector quality strategies can be said to fall into two categories.

On the one hand, there are the neo-Taylorist *compliance* models of quality control, which are based on monitoring and appraisal and are outcomes-driven. Compliance models define quality as 'fitness for purpose'. They involve the specification of standards and the institution of formal systems of quality control to ensure that products conform to these standards. Compliance models, therefore, tend to be associated with the development of elaborate systems of performance measurement and external audits, and are characterised by routinisation and standardisation.

A very different approach to quality assurance in the private sector is the post-Taylorist *consumerist* (or total quality management) process-driven model, where quality is understood as meaning pleasing or satisfying the consumer (Gaster 1999). Here there is an emphasis on strong leadership, vision and employee involvement. Consumerist organisations are customer driven. They emphasise flexibility and responsiveness rather than standardisation. Some have argued that this approach is potentially empowering for consumers, because it is customer-centred, and that it is potentially empowering for workers, because it is based on the belief that 'quality improvement . . . can only be achieved if all staff are equally involved, committed and given the space and responsibility to make decisions' (Kirkpatrick and Martinez-Lucio 1995), although, as one observer of total quality management (TQM) in both private and public sectors has commented, that potential does not seem to have been realised:

> The private sector experience of TQM is instructive: despite very strong, almost missionary beliefs about its efficacy, it has failed again and again . . . It is generally implemented top-down, it is highly managerial, and it lacks active consumer participation.
>
> (Gaster 1999)

In education, the Conservatives borrowed selectively from both models. So, on the one hand, as we saw in Chapter 1, markets in schooling were justified on the grounds that they would empower consumers in relation to producers. On the other hand, we also saw that the market could not be trusted fully to ensure that school quality was of the right type. For example, whilst the 'industrial trainers' within the Conservative Party wanted schools to promote the kinds of attitudes and skills they believed were appropriate for an advanced economy, the neo-conservatives wanted to ensure that schools promoted the 'traditional' values of respect for the family, private property and authority. So, at the same time as introducing a market in education, the Conservatives borrowed from the compliance school of quality control, an emphasis on the specification and monitoring of standards. This was to be achieved through the national curriculum, regular testing of students, performance tables and Ofsted. We have seen in Part I of this book that the emphasis on compliance, and the managerial control that went with it, effectively ruled out the possibility of schools introducing the more empowering aspects of the consumerist model of quality.

Broadly speaking, New Labour has sought to retain the quality edifice built up by the Conservatives. Crucially – despite the rhetorical emphasis on collaboration, partnership and community – market forces have been preserved, with resources still distributed to schools primarily on a *per capita* basis. Indeed, in some respects marketisation has been reinforced, for example, by the creation of more specialist schools to diversify the market choice available to (some) parents and children. And New Labour has extended some of the privatising elements of the Conservative reforms. Although it is phasing out the Assisted Places Scheme – which involves the use of state funds to subsidise places in private schools – the government is seeking to further 'diversify' provision in other ways. For example, it is encouraging more private sector involvement in the running of schools, through the Private Finance Initiative,[22] Education Action Zones (EAZs)[23] and City Academies.[24] It is also promoting the 'out-sourcing' of LEA services to private companies and the establishment of fixed-term 'standards contracts' allowing private companies, as well as charities, churches and other religious organisations, to take over the running of schools from LEAs. A further diminution in the role of the LEA is threatened by what appears to be an increasing trend for central government to fund schools directly.[25]

22 The Private Finance Initiative (PFI) was first introduced by the Conservatives in 1992. It is a scheme whereby private investment is used to build and operate public facilities, like schools and hospitals, and these are then leased back to the public sector. In the long run this method of funding public services tends to cost more – because private companies usually have to pay higher interest rates for borrowing money than the state. However, it costs less for the state initially, because the state pays back the money over periods of between 20 and 60 years (Cohen 1999: 31). As Ling comments, this 'allows political gains to be made today and the costs imposed on future governments' (Ling 2000: 97).

23 The EAZs initiative was introduced in 1998 as a strategy for raising educational standards in areas of social disadvantage. An EAZ consists of around 20 schools, usually around three secondaries and their feeder primaries. Each zone receives up to £750,000 per year from the government over a three to five year period and is expected to raise a further £250,000 per year from other (private) sources – in cash or 'kind'. The government is keen for zones to be run by private sponsors but the vast majority of the current 73 zones up and running are LEA led.

24 The City Academies initiative, announced in March 2000, is modelled on the Conservative government's City Technology Colleges policy. It enables private and voluntary sector organisations to establish and run urban schools independently of LEAs.

25 The March 2000 Budget put £300 million directly into schools, bypassing the local authorities.

At the same time, New Labour have warmly embraced and extended the compliance-based elements of the Conservatives' policies. They are actively promoting performance monitoring and target setting in schools and local authorities. And, as a means of enforcing even stricter compliance to their conceptions of quality, the government has introduced performance-related pay (PRP) for teachers. New Labour has also adopted with gusto the contract model of resource allocation, whereby schools wanting to gain funds in addition to what they get from the LEA's per capita-based formula must bid for money that is attached to particular government initiatives – for example, 'specialist schools', 'early excellence centres', 'family literacy schemes' and 'work-related learning' – all of which are only funded for a limited period. This targeted and time-limited approach to funding is viewed as an effective means of ensuring that schools and LEAs comply with centrally-approved ideas about what works best but, as I argue below, it has potentially inequitable consequences.

New Labour has also embraced Ofsted's inspection regime, which it sees as an essential tool for rooting out 'defective' teachers, schools and LEAs. And of course Ofsted is only one of a number of regulatory bodies that now have a responsibility for overseeing some aspect of quality in the schools sector. As Hood *et al.* (1999) point out, schools in England have been 'subject to multiple, sometimes overlapping overseers' (1999: 142). In addition to Ofsted, there is the Qualifications and Curriculum Authority, which regulates the national curriculum and oversees assessment, and the Teacher Training Agency, responsible for the funding and quality control of teacher education. In addition, LEAs still act as 'first-line regulators' (Hood *et al.* 1999) of schools and in certain circumstances they can resume control of a school where it is deemed to be failing. Under Conservative governments, the Audit Commission already had a responsibility for evaluating the 'economy', 'efficiency' and 'effectiveness' of schools as part of its broader remit to oversee local government. But New Labour has conferred an additional duty upon the Audit Commission. Now, in conjunction with Ofsted, it must conduct regular inspections of LEAs. New Labour has also added to this assortment of overseers, setting up the Standards and Effectiveness Unit within the DfEE (now DfES – Department for Education and Skills), which, as Hood *et al.* point out, has 'taken a keen interest in the performance of LEAs as monitors of school performance' (1999: 145).

This stepping up of surveillance by New Labour appears to represent a concerted effort to secure a reformation of teachers and teaching practices. The Standards and Effectiveness Unit is headed up by

Professor Michael Barber, a former adviser to the Labour Party and author of *The Learning Game: Arguments for an Education Revolution* (1996), a text that has had a significant influence on New Labour policy-making in education. In Chapter 1, I cited Barber's dismissal of arguments that the causes of educational underattainment are primarily structural and his belief that it is teachers and schools who bear the brunt of responsibility for school failure. This view has come to dominate New Labour thinking despite contrary evidence (Mortimore and Whitty 1997; Thrupp 1999).

Thus, in the government's diagnosis of the 'crisis of schooling', teachers are part of the problem, as they were for the Conservative reformers of the 1980s and 1990s. Apparently steeped in reactionary values, teachers, alongside other public-sector workers, are seen to represent the forces of conservatism (an epithet that New Labour has used to deride what it calls extremists of the left and the right) – resistant to change, inflexible and in need of modernisation and discipline (Carvel and Brindle 1999: 3). It is perhaps the perceived recalcitrance of teachers more than anything which explains the strength of New Labour's commitment to 'continuous improvement' via a hard-edged inspection regime, the extensive use of performance indicators and targets, PRP and the rooting out of headteachers who are resistant to 'modernisation'.[26] These strategies are, at least in part, designed to secure the installation of traditional pedagogic approaches in schools. These are deemed to be more effective both at combating disadvantage in education and preparing children for the world of work than the more child-centred methods preferred by many teachers, especially those working in primary schools. Whilst, as we have seen in earlier chapters, Conservative policies of national testing, league tables, the regular inspection of schools by Ofsted and the reduction of the continuous assessment component of GCSEs combined to encourage conservative pedagogies in schools, Conservative governments did not intervene directly to shape schools' pedagogical strategies. New Labour has taken that step, introducing the highly prescriptive and teacher-centred literacy and numeracy hours in primary schools, a policy which has recently been extended to secondaries. New Labour also believes that 'setting should be the norm in secondary schools' and that 'it is worth considering in primary schools' (DfEE 1997c: 38).

26 In 1999, New Labour was reported as having set aside £10 million for the early retirement of headteachers who were deemed 'unlikely to adapt well to carrying forward the major changes envisaged in improving education' (Bunting 1999: 1).

But, for New Labour, teachers are not the only obstacle to the creation of a 'modern' education system which is equipped to sustain the 'modern dynamic economy' that New Labour wants to build (Blair 1998). The so-called wastage of human capital is seen to be especially significant in 'disadvantaged' areas where there are low levels of academic attainment and high rates of absenteeism and exclusion from school. And parents (or at least some working-class parents), as well as teachers, are held to be to blame here. So, as well as tightening up the regulation of teachers, New Labour is also attempting to regulate parents more effectively by making them more responsible and, if necessary, forcing them to share the values upon which 'strong communities' are seen to depend. As Blair has argued:

> Strong communities depend on shared values and a recognition of the rights and duties of citizenship – not just the duty to pay taxes and obey the law, but the obligation to bring up children as competent, responsible citizens, and to support those – such as teachers – who are employed by the state in the task. In the past we have tended to take such duties for granted. But where they are neglected, we should not hesitate to encourage and even enforce them, as we are seeking to do with initiatives such as our 'home-school contracts' between schools and parents.
>
> (Blair 1998: 12)

Thus, there is a clear emphasis within New Labour's third way agenda for education on what Nikolas Rose (1996) has called 'responsibilisation' – the process of inculcating a culture of self-discipline or self-surveillance amongst welfare subjects. Responsibilisation appears to be a strategy that is being pursued with even more vigour by New Labour than it was by its Conservative predecessors.[27] Under New Labour, schools are required to produce home-school agreements, the government has specified the precise numbers of hours of homework students are expected to do and that parents are expected to supervise, and it has set up 'family learning schemes' and programmes for 'better' parenting. Such moral authoritarian strategies, often couched in the communitarian language of 'social capital building', can be viewed as part of a broader 'campaign' to tackle social exclusion

---

27 Although it is important to remember that responsibilisation was also a key Conservative strategy, particularly evident in the *Parents' Charter* (DES 1991; DFE 1994a) and in the DFE's approach to 'Pupils with Problems' (DFE 1994b; Evans and Vincent 1997).

by reforming the attitudes and behaviour of the socially excluded themselves, rather than by addressing the structural causes of exclusion – for example, the unequal distribution of adequately remunerated jobs. New Labour views the latter as a consequence of global capitalism that cannot – or should not – be bucked (Hall 1998). Thus, the state under New Labour appears to be intensifying its focus on individual behaviour, the family and issues of morality, as it simultaneously absolves itself of responsibility for the macro-economic, infrastructural conditions that actually induce – and also have the potential to reduce – social exclusion in the first place.[28]

Clearly then, although there are differences in emphasis and presentation, there are significant continuities between New Right and New Labour policies for education around the neo-liberal/authoritarian nexus – evident in shared propensities towards the 'quality' strategies of 'choice' and 'diversity', privatisation, standardisation and regulation, as well as responsibilisation and pedagogic traditionalism. Yet alongside these neo-liberal and authoritarian tendencies, there are other – apparently more humanistic – strands of New Labour's agenda for schools. There is at least a rhetorical valuing of (some) diverse cultural identities, 'citizenship education', equality of opportunity and more open, responsive and democratic government. For example, in his Fabian pamphlet on the third way, Blair argued that 'the democratic impulse needs to be strengthened by finding new ways to enable citizens to share in decision making that affects them' (Blair 1998: 15). And New Labour's *Modernising Government* White Paper was very critical of the failure of public services in the past to involve and meet the needs of different groups in society:

> There is no such thing as a 'typical' citizen. People's needs and concerns differ . . . some of these concerns have not been given sufficient recognition in the past. We must understand the needs of all people and respond to them.
>
> (Cabinet Office 1999: 4)

These more humanistic elements of third way thinking were reflected in the government's 1999 revision of the national curriculum for England, which, for the first time, included 'citizenship' as part of the statutory curriculum, and in the revised framework for the inspection

---

28 As Judy Hirst (2000: 24) observes in relation to employment policy, the focus on building individuals' 'capacity' through counselling and training is cheaper than major infrastructural, job-creating programmes.

of schools (Ofsted 2000). The revised curriculum begins with a statement of values the government says it wishes to promote in education:

> Foremost is a belief in education, at home and at school, as a route to the spiritual, moral, social, cultural, physical and mental development, and thus the well-being, of the individual. Education is also a route to equality of opportunity for all, a healthy and just democracy, a productive economy, and sustainable development. Education should reflect the enduring values that contribute to these ends. These include valuing ourselves, our families and other relationships, the wider groups to which we belong, the diversity in our society and the environment in which we live. Education should also reaffirm our commitment to the virtues of truth, justice, honesty, trust and a sense of duty.
>
> (QCA/DfEE 1999a)

At least some of these values are reflected in the post-Macpherson revised handbook for school inspections. This instructs inspectors to report on: 'the extent to which pupils work in an atmosphere free from oppressive behaviour, including bullying, sexism and racism'; and 'how far pupils recognise, understand and respect different values and beliefs, attitudes, and social and cultural traditions' (Ofsted 2000).

There is also an increased emphasis in New Labour discourse on partnership and participation in the organisation of school provision, with the government having introduced a number of policies that might be described as associationalist; that is, concerned to facilitate new forms of civic association and collective responsibility. Strategies of associationalism are evident in: the expectation that specialist schools will be established within 'collaborative', 'new learning' networks; the introduction of parent representatives on local authority education committees;[29] and the inclusion of representatives of community groups, alongside school, business and LEA representatives, on the Education Action Forums that are meant to run EAZs.

Finally, there is an emphasis on additional funding for schools, particularly in areas designated as socially disadvantaged, in order to combat 'social exclusion', through the Excellence in Cities, EAZ

---

29 However, this particular associational strategy has been significantly undermined by New Labour's local government reforms: these require councils to establish cabinet-style executives with elected mayors, leaders or council managers in place of the traditional committee structure which gave representatives of various local constituencies an opportunity to participate in local decision making.

and City Academies initiatives. This appears to mark a distinct shift from Conservative policies. As we have seen in earlier chapters, although redistribution was not a prominent discourse under the Conservatives, significant redistributions did occur, mainly via the market and grant-maintained schools mechanisms. But these were redistributions that tended to favour the most advantaged students and discriminate against working-class families and particular racialised groups. Contemporary policy rhetoric suggests that New Labour wants to reverse this trend.

So it is apparent that there are tensions within New Labour's educational agenda. On the one hand, the government is committed to a model of reform that emphasises markets, compliance, standardisation, responsibilisation and pedagogic traditionalism, and that is based on a belief in the superiority of private-sector management practices. On the other hand, it aligns itself with the need to combat social exclusion, widen participation in the running of schools and to promote, through its proposals for 'citizenship education', the values of democracy, social justice and respect for cultural diversity.

As with the tensions evident in New Right policy, we should not be surprised by the contradictory nature of New Labour's agenda. For policy programmes are inherently complex and contradictory: they tend to be shaped by a range of different, and often conflicting, political and economic interests, and they are designed to simultaneously resolve a variety of problems, crises or instabilities, each of which require different solutions. Thus, as I argued in Chapter 6, the Conservative strategies of marketisation and managerialisation appeared increasingly unable to simultaneously resolve perceived problems of capital accumulation, social control and legitimacy. Instead, the policies had begun to generate a stressed workforce, a crisis in teacher recruitment and retention, polarised and segregated schooling, the increased exploitation and marginalisation of teachers and students, and culturally imperialist curricular practices. Taken together – and in conjunction with the growth in inequalities of health and income produced by the economic and social policies of successive Conservative governments (Hills 1995; Piachaud 1999) – these developments created the possibility of widespread social discontent, particularly in urban areas where they were experienced in an intensified form. As we saw in Chapter 6, these developments could also be viewed as representing a potential threat to the ability of the education system to adequately support processes of capital accumulation. For teacher stress and shortages along with increased polarisation mitigate against the production of the highly-skilled workforce that is seen to be necessary if

Britain is to be successful in transforming itself into a high-wage, high-productivity economy. Finally, these developments threatened a potential crisis of legitimacy, as large sections of the public became increasingly sceptical about the ability of public-sector markets to deliver the widespread choice, diversity and quality that had been promised. Thus, Conservative policies appear to have reproduced the problems they were designed to solve, albeit in new forms.

These are the very problems that, in turn, New Labour policies appear to be aimed at resolving. Thus, on the one hand, we are seeing an intensification of what Ozga (2000) has dubbed 'the economising of education', where what goes on in schools is increasingly shaped by the narrowly perceived requirements of the economy – to the extent that, as one commentator has recently put it, childhood becomes a training for employment (Bunting 2000). For New Labour, 'human and intellectual capital' is 'the main source of value and competitive advantage in the modern economy' (Blair 1998: 10). Thus, according to New Labour logic, priority needs to be given to a system of education and training within which teachers and parents are even more tightly controlled than they were under the Conservatives. And there needs to be a more specific targeting of resources upon those activities and approaches that are believed to produce human and intellectual capital of the right kind. At the same time, the more humanistic elements of New Labour's education agenda appear to be aimed at remedying other 'design flaws' of Conservative policies. In particular, it would seem that they are aimed at circumventing the threats to social control and legitimacy prompted by the increase in exclusion, polarisation and fragmentation associated with marketisation.

Of course, there may also be other pressures at work as well. In Chapter 6, I quoted Dale's (1989) comment that not everything the state does can be explained in terms of the problems of the state or the education system. Thus, for example, New Labour's first Secretary of State for Education, David Blunkett's former incarnation as a key player in the New Left urban politics of the 1980s may be significant. Despite his dirigiste orientation in government, as leader of Sheffield Council, Blunkett had been a vocal advocate for the democratisation of local politics and this should not be discounted altogether as an influence on the more associationalist elements of New Labour's agenda for education.

Later in the chapter, I want to consider the likely success of New Labour's third way in remedying the 'design flaws' of Conservative post-welfarism in education. But first, I want to deal with the consequences of this contradictory and complex mix of neo-liberal, authoritarian and humanistic policies for social justice. I want to begin by focusing on its distributional implications before going on to consider issues of relational justice (see Chapter 7).

Distributional implications

As I suggested in the previous section, New Labour policies suggest a commitment to a degree of *progressive* redistribution. However, New Labour's stance on redistribution is complex and this is partly due to what might be termed the politics of electability. On the one hand, the government does not want to alienate those sections of the population that are believed to constitute 'middle England' by appearing profligate and to be increasing the tax 'burden'. On the other hand, there appears to be a recognition that, although it wants to pay less tax, 'middle England' is also apparently concerned about under-investment in public services, particularly health and education. And the government has the added pressure of wanting to retain the support of the so-called Labour 'heartlands'. Thus, New Labour policy makers and spin doctors have had to perform a precarious balancing act, which has resulted in them refusing to use the word redistribution, whilst announcing what is claimed to be significant additional investment in education.

To make matters more complicated, there is some dispute about whether the extent of additional investment is as great as the government claims (Davies 2000; Denny and Elliott 2001). However, even if we take New Labour figures at face value, the degree of redistribution appears fairly limited. For example, each EAZ containing approximately 20 schools, receives only around £1 million per year (three-quarters of which comes from the state and the other quarter from private sources – in cash or kind). This is significantly less than the annual income of an average-sized secondary school. And the smaller-sized infant classes, which the government claimed to be funding by the phasing out of the Assisted Places Scheme, have been accompanied by an increase in class sizes for older age groups.[30]

---

30 Figures published by the DfEE in April 2000 indicated that, whilst the government was on target to meet its pledge that no 5, 6 or 7-year-old would be taught in a class of 31 or more by September 2001, the number of secondary school pupils in classes of over 30 had more than doubled since 1990 and had risen by nearly 20 per cent since 1998 (cited in Thornton 2000: 4).

There are a number of other reasons – aside, that is, from the relatively limited quantity of funds being redistributed – why we may have to be sceptical about how extensively redistributive New Labour's education policies are. First, we have seen that New Labour remains committed to the principles of choice and competition. Given this support for markets in education, it is difficult to see how the targeting of limited additional resources on specific schools through the Excellence in Cities, EAZs, specialist schools and City Academies policies will be able to interrupt the processes of segregation and polarisation that markets seem to produce. It is conceivable that some schools may 'improve' as a consequence of additional resources. But the likelihood is that within the competitive local market environments that New Labour are retaining, school 'improvement' will depend upon schools becoming more popular with the kinds of 'able' or 'motivated' students likely to perform well in their end of Key Stage tests (standard assessment tasks or SATs) and GCSEs. Hence, the improvement of schools is likely to continue to be at the expense of those neighbouring schools who lose their more 'valuable' students to the improving schools. For, as I argued in Chapter 5, within a marketised education system, 'good' management may be able to produce a redistribution of students amongst schools but it cannot address the root causes of educational underattainment.

Second, the managerial practice of target setting, which New Labour is encouraging, is, if we are to extrapolate from past evidence, likely to lead teachers to focus on those students just below the required level, rather than the lowest-achieving students (Gewirtz *et al.* 1995; Gillborn and Youdell 1999). And, traditional pedagogical practices, like setting and whole class teaching, which are central features of the literacy and numeracy strategies, also have the potential to further a *regressive* redistribution of resources. I am referring here to a redistribution *away* from students deemed to be 'less able' and, in the case of setting, students from working-class families, especially boys and particular racialised groups, towards those 'able', middle-class, mainly white students who most benefit from setted regimes and whole-class teaching (Oakes 1990; Hallam and Toutounji 1996; Slavin 1996; Sukhnandan and Lee 1998). Furthermore, the lowering of class sizes in primary schools to 30 students or fewer may have the perverse effect of redistributing resources in favour of schools in relatively advantaged areas (since inner-city schools are more likely to have lower rolls and therefore smaller class sizes to begin with).

Third, as we have seen, a rapidly increasing proportion of funds for education is being distributed on a contract basis. This involves schools, LEAs – or, in the case of EAZs, 'partnerships' – having to bid for money from the DfES's 'Standards Fund' and other sources, like the Single Regeneration Budget and the lottery-based New Opportunities Fund. As noted above, these various sources of funding are time limited and tied to specific projects. They also usually require 'matched' funding from the LEA. This has potentially serious consequences both for continuity of provision and for equity. Mike Eastwood's (1999) comments on the impact of the National Opportunities Fund's bidding system on charities are equally applicable to schools. He describes a situation in which 'charities wander from funder to funder, repackaging old work as though it were new, promising financial sustainability and tangible benefits within an impossibly short period of time' (Eastwood 1999: xxv). And because, within the bidding system, money is distributed on the basis of an assessment of the quality of the bid, there is no guarantee that resources are being directed where they are most needed. One distinct possibility is that resources will accumulate in those areas and institutions with the most skilled bidders. Indeed, research undertaken by a former education spokesperson for the Liberal Democrats, Don Foster MP, found that better-off authorities tended to be more successful in accruing Standards Fund money because they had more staff and resources to prepare bids (cited in Davies 2000: 11). And a successful bid from one source tends to attract further funding from other sources, leading to an even greater disparity between successful and unsuccessful bidders. Moreover, significant amounts of LEA money, which could be spent directly on teachers and classroom resources, are being diverted to paying for the consultants who are employed to write the numerous bids, not all of which are successful. Nick Davies has reported that 'during Mr Blunkett's first two years [as Secretary of State for Education] there were 25,353 bids but only 8,972 were successful. Oxfordshire made 1,015 bids and saw 1,002 of them fail. Blackpool put in 212 bids and succeeded with only 10' (Davies 2000: 11). The bidding process also consumes significant quantities of headteacher and senior management time (Mountfield and Eastwood 2000). Furthermore, because LEAs have to 'match' half of the value of the Standards Fund money they receive, they are forced to divert resources from their delegated schools budget to supplement targeted Standards Fund projects (Davies 2000: 11). Research commissioned by the Directory for Social Change has found growing disparities on a worrying scale between schools in disadvantaged areas and those in better-off districts in terms of success in accessing funding from businesses and charities (Mountfield and Eastwood 2000).

Finally, New Labour is committed to the involvement of the private sector in the running of schools, which may well exacerbate the regressive distribution of resources that market forces produce. For the likelihood is that private companies, motivated by profit and the desire to demonstrate success, will be reluctant to spend resources on those students deemed to be least motivated and underattaining. In arguing for the value of private sector involvement in the provision of schooling, the government has pointed to the academic success of city technology colleges (CTCs), which are run by governing bodies upon which commercial sponsors have built-in majorities. Indeed, the City Academies initiative is explicitly modelled on the CTC programme. Rarely is it mentioned, however, that whilst the CTCs may have to take children across the whole measured ability range, they are able to select students (and their parents) by interview and on the basis of aptitude and commitment to staying on in education until age 18. Thus, whilst CTCs may appear to take a representative cross section of students from different class and ethnic backgrounds, they are able to select those students deemed to be the most motivated and potentially 'high-performing', whilst rejecting those viewed as disaffected, damaged or really disadvantaged. It is, therefore, difficult to see how New Labour policies are going to disrupt the processes of differential valuing generated by Conservative reforms. As long as a market system of resource allocation is in place, students will continue to be valued and selected according to how much they contribute to a school's image and performance. And this will disproportionately disadvantage those from economically marginalised populations and particular racialised groupings.

Relational implications

As we saw in Chapter 7, the differential valuing of students, which markets and selection generate, not only has consequences for distributional justice but for relational justice too. Differential valuing and the polarisation that results from it perpetuate the injustices of marginalisation and powerlessness experienced by those groups of students who are least valued and who, as a consequence, are ghettoised in the least-resourced schools. In Chapter 7, I also suggested that the treatment of students as commodities in the marketplace, to be attracted or rejected according to what they can offer the school, represents a form of exploitation. The analysis in the previous section suggests that third way policies are unlikely to disrupt these processes of commodification, differential valuing and polarisation. And, hence, we might reasonably conclude that the injustices of exploitation, marginalisation and powerlessness that some groups of students appear to be experiencing, as a consequence of Conservative post-welfarism, will be perpetuated by New Labour so long as the *per capita* mechanism and the preoccupation with narrow conceptions of performance remain intact.

I now want to consider three additional aspects of the relational implications of New Labour's third way agenda by focusing on its consequences for parental participation in education, teachers' work and the curriculum. Particular emphasis is given to the curricular implications of the reforms, as this is where the tensions between New Labour's neo-liberal authoritarianism and its humanism are most apparent.

Parental participation

In New Labour's presentation of their policies, parents are not simply consumers. As noted above, the government has further increased parental representation on governing bodies, has introduced the requirement that parents be represented on local authority education committees (but see Footnote 29) and has included parent representatives on the forums that are meant to run EAZs. David Halpin (1999) has suggested that these Education Action Forums represent an investment in social capital and that they could prefigure a revivified civil society within which parents and other community members are 'empowered' to take more control of local services (see also Whitty 1998). However, I want to suggest that this kind of analysis obscures the potentially damaging implications of increased private sector involvement in the running of schools and overlooks the potentially exclusionary nature of New Labour's experiments in social capital building. For, as those working within feminist and Foucauldian perspectives have pointed out, practices designed to promote social capital have the potential to exclude as well as include (Campbell 1995; Hughes and Mooney 1998). In particular, it is highly questionable how far the private companies involved in the running of schools will want to cede control to parents and other community groups in any meaningful way where this might conflict with the companies' own commercial interests. And where private companies are given a *central role* in the running of schools, there are likely to be a number of voices and interests that are excluded or at least marginalised: for example, teachers opposed to a further intensification of their work and to changes in their terms and conditions; parents opposed to the fact that sponsoring companies might direct advertising at their children who are effectively a captive audience when at school; those opposed to the ethical practices of some of the companies involved; and those opposed to *any* involvement of private companies in the provision of education. Moreover, whilst New Labour strategies of individual 'responsibilisation', like family literacy or inter-generational learning schemes, may have the potential to facilitate perceptions of inclusivity amongst members of previously excluded social groups, these strategies also have the potential to make people feel they are being constructed as a problem, hence exacerbating their perceptions of marginality. And, most crucially, such strategies do not deal with the *causes* of social exclusion, which New Labour blames on the forces of globalisation that cannot or should not be meddled with (Hall 1998).

In general, it would seem that New Labour has a very narrow conception of parental participation in education. This seems to have been largely reduced to an individualised conception of involvement. For New Labour, parental involvement seems to mean equipping parents, and where necessary forcing them, to be more responsible for and involved in their own children's learning, for example, through family learning schemes, home-school agreements, working with their children at home following school and DfES guidelines, and harsh penalties for truancy – a manifestation of what New Labour's first Secretary of State for Education, David Blunkett, has called 'tough love'. So it would seem that New Labour are happy to encourage citizens to share in limited forms of decision making but only on condition that they behave in what are deemed to be responsible ways. Effectively, this means endorsing what New Labour wants, which in some instances includes parents being made to accept a business 'take-over' of their schools.

Teachers' work

In the previous chapter, I argued that the Conservative government's post-welfarist policies appeared to be contributing to the exploitation of teachers. I suggested this was because teachers were having to work harder to serve other people's interests whilst at the same time deriving less personal satisfaction from their work. It seems to me that under New Labour this trend will be exacerbated, as schools and the teaching profession are 'modernised' in the interests of the 'dynamic, modern economy' that the government wants to create.

First, the high degree of surveillance of teachers generated by Conservative policies is, as we have seen, being intensified under New

Labour through the retention of the Ofsted regime of inspections, national testing and examination league tables, the increase in the proportion of funds for education distributed on a contract basis, the insistence on more target setting and performance monitoring in schools and the introduction of PRP. Second, the introduction of PRP is likely to intensify the pressure on teachers to increase productivity. Third, teaching is being further technicised and routinised, and the scope for autonomous teacher activity further limited. This is being achieved by the introduction of the literacy and numeracy hours, which prescribe the content of teaching in these areas, and by the arrangements for PRP, within which teachers will be competing with each other for salary increments on the basis of narrow prescriptions of what counts as good teaching. John Smyth and Geoffrey Shacklock's (1998) study of the Australian Advanced Skills Teachers' initiative has shown how such performance-related schemes contribute to a fragmentation and routinisation of teachers' work and make it more amenable to tight managerial control. Such routinisation is likely to be exacerbated by New Labour's introduction of optional annual tests, which schools can volunteer for in addition to the end of key-stage tests. Increasing numbers of schools are volunteering for these tests in order to facilitate the assessment of teacher performance for PRP purposes (Henry 2000). This is a classic example of how the discourse of performativity works to change what goes on inside schools, as school processes and practices become increasingly shaped by the requirements of performance-monitoring systems rather than the interests of students. Fourth, tensions between staff will inevitably be produced or intensified by the introduction of PRP, whereby teachers' salaries are at least partly determined by the judgements that their colleagues make of them and their work.[31] This is likely to further undermine the kinds of collaborative relationships which for many teachers are a fundamental component of what makes their work fulfilling.

But to what extent will teachers be financially compensated for the likely further diminution of collegiality in schools and the increased intensification, routinisation and regulation of their work? New Labour's policies on teachers' pay may lead to improvements for those in managerial positions, those successful in gaining the new Advanced Skills Teachers' (AST) (or Super Teacher) status, those

---

31 Heads of department and senior teachers now have a duty written in to their contracts to assist the headteacher in carrying out 'threshold assessments' of other teachers (Barnard and Henry 2000: 1).

passing the 'performance threshold' (which entitles them to move on to a higher pay scale) and those accepted onto the 'fast-track' scheme designed 'to attract able graduates' and 'move outstanding teachers quickly through the profession' (DfEE 1998). But these policies seem unlikely to result in significant pay increases for the 'ordinary' classroom teacher. In addition, as Ozga has noted, PRP carries with it the risk of exacerbating existing tendencies towards discrimination against women 'who consistently undersell themselves in such self-promoting systems' and who are 'more likely then men to spend time and effort on unremarked tasks that do not carry weight in the appraisal process' (Ozga 2000: 231). Furthermore, studies of PRP schemes in a range of public services have pointed to perceptions amongst affected staff that PRP is open to abuse, highly personalised and used by management to reward their favourites and that it discriminates against part timers and members of ethnic minorities (Waine 2000).

New Labour's policies also have important implications for classroom assistants. The Green Paper, *Teachers: Meeting the Challenge of Change* (DfEE 1998), suggested that the number of teaching assistant posts would be increased by at least 20,000 by the year 2002 but it is yet to be seen how successful the campaigns for improving the pay and status of classroom assistants and nursery nurses in schools will be.

The curriculum

The instrumentalism and narrowness of focus of Conservative post-welfarism can be viewed as having promoted cultural imperialism, in part, by routinely subjecting many young people to curricular practices that neither engage with nor value their own cultural identities (see Chapter 7). Under New Labour, the official view of good teaching continues to be synonymous with Ofsted's view, with its emphasis on outcomes and a utilitarian, test-oriented, didactic approach. As Peter Woods and Bob Jeffrey (1998) argue in relation to primary education, Ofsted's transmissional and hierarchical model of teaching is in direct opposition to that of most primary teachers who 'believe in holistic, integrated knowledge, child-centred teaching methods, a measure of professional autonomy, continuous and formative assessment and collaborative teaching cultures' (1998: 548).

Whilst the contrast between official versions of quality and teachers' own versions of quality are perhaps most stark in the primary school, the pedagogic traditionalism espoused by New Labour is also alien to practices and approaches preferred by many secondary school teachers.

For example, Ken Jones (1999) writes of how from the 1970s to the early 1990s many English teachers refashioned the curriculum in order that it should engage with the experiences, language and culture that students brought with them to the classroom. In this way, the curriculum could be made relevant, accessible and enjoyable. Rather than segregating students in hierarchically ordered ability groups on the basis of students' 'degree of comfort with quite narrow cultural forms' (Jones 1999: 49), these teachers enabled students to engage with what they knew and what they could do, and thereby managed to displace the ethno-centric tendencies in the traditionalist English curriculum. At the same time critical reflection was encouraged. What this meant was that whilst the knowledge and experience of students was validated, students were at the same time asked to question that knowledge 'in the process of making sense of and responding to a particular text' (Jones 1999: 53). This approach 'draws from experience, but does not hesitate to cross its boundaries' (Jones 1999: 53). However, as Jones argues, these skills of critical reflection are currently undervalued within official quality discourses, as is the importance of engaging with students' own interests and cultural experiences. A similar story can be told about other areas of the curriculum (Hill and Cole 1999).[32]

The slimming down of the national curriculum by New Labour through the reduction of statutory requirements and prescriptive detail announced in 1999 may well allow greater room for professional autonomy and greater responsiveness to students' needs and interests, as is suggested in the government's revised national curriculum. The stated aims for the revised national curriculum include the economistic, instrumentalist goals of equipping students 'for their future lives as workers' and 'consumers' and 'preparing them for the next steps in their education, training and employment'. They also include 'responsibilising' goals, such as encouraging in students a recognition of the importance of leading 'a healthy lifestyle and keeping themselves and others safe'. But these are combined with the more humanistic aims of:

---

32 For example, Peter Bailey has argued that, as is the case with English teaching, the official approach to maths in the secondary school prioritises the transmission of an ethno-centric body of knowledge and marginalises alternative approaches. As teachers are increasingly being judged on how their students perform in GSCEs, more time is being devoted to practising for exams (Bailey 1999: 63–4). And there is less room for teaching that helps students make connections between their own informal knowledge and new knowledge or which helps students 'to use their mathematics to understand and play an active part in the world' (Bailey 1999: 59; see also Boaler 1994).

- developing 'enjoyment of, and commitment to, learning'
- building on 'pupils' strengths, interests and experiences'
- contributing 'to the development of pupils' sense of identity through knowledge and understanding of the spiritual, moral, social and cultural heritages of Britain's diverse society and of the local, national, European, Commonwealth and global dimensions of their lives'
- enabling 'pupils to think creatively and critically, to solve problems and to make a difference for the better'
- developing students' 'knowledge, understanding and appreciation of their own and different beliefs and cultures, and how these influence individuals and societies'
- developing 'pupils' integrity and autonomy'
- helping them to be 'caring citizens capable of contributing to the development of a just society'
- promoting 'equal opportunities'
- enabling 'pupils to challenge discrimination and stereotyping'
- developing 'their awareness and understanding of, and respect for, the environments in which they live'
- promoting 'pupils' self-esteem and emotional well-being'
- helping 'them to form and maintain worthwhile and satisfying relationships, based on respect for themselves and for others, at home, school, work and in the community'
- developing their ability 'to relate to others and work for the common good'.

(QCA/DfEE 1999a)

The new national curriculum was published shortly after the Macpherson Report (Macpherson 1999), which had recommended that the national curriculum be revised to emphasise a valuing of cultural diversity and the prevention of racism. However, whilst the revised national curriculum includes several references to 'valuing cultural diversity', the issue of racism is altogether absent from the citizenship curriculum and, as Audrey Osler has pointed out, there is nothing which begins to address institutionalised racism (Osler 1999: 8–9), despite Macpherson's recommendation that schools tackle this issue.[33] But even the more limited commitment to valuing cultural diversity is in tension with the neo-liberal and authoritarian elements of New

33 Although it is significant that the revised handbook for school inspections does require inspectors to consider 'how far pupils are able to work in an atmosphere . . . free from sexism and racism' (Ofsted 2000).

Labour's third way agenda. And it may well be that the neo-liberal and authoritarian elements will prevent the more humanistic curriculum aims from being realised. I want to conclude this section by drawing attention to four ways in which this may be the case.

First, the government has stated that it wants the curriculum to promote equal opportunities and enable pupils to challenge discrimination and stereotyping through the provision of 'citizenship education'. Yet, the market and compliance models of quality control are encouraging schools to adopt practices of setting and selection. And, as so much research demonstrates, these practices facilitate both discrimination and stereotyping (e.g., Oakes 1990; Hallam and Toutounji 1996; Slavin 1996; Boaler 1997a; Sukhnandan and Lee 1998). It is also important to note that, whilst New Labour have abolished grant-maintained school status, they have retained the status differentials amongst schools, by giving former grant-maintained schools the option of calling themselves 'foundation' rather than 'community' schools. New Labour policies are, therefore, likely to create the very environments which are generating the kinds of exclusionary and hierarchical practices that the government claims it wants the curriculum to combat. So it will be very difficult for teachers to educate children about the damaging consequences of discrimination and stereotyping without them also challenging the hierarchical, socially segregated and discriminatory contexts within which learning is likely to be increasingly set.

Second, as I have already sought to demonstrate, it is difficult to see how a compliance-based approach to quality is compatible with pedagogical practices that foster autonomy and creativity, and that engage with students' own cultural experiences. Labour's enthusiasm for target setting and PRP is only likely to intensify the focus in schools on those activities that can be, and are being, measured and on those things teachers are going to be rewarded for. Autonomy, creativity and critical thinking are not easily amenable to measurement. And nor does it seem that they are valued in the current system of assessment upon which teachers' pay will be partly based.

Third, schools, through 'citizenship education', are meant to be giving students the knowledge, understanding and skills to enable them to participate in society as 'active citizens of democracy' and to contribute to the development of a just society. Schools are also meant to inculcate 'a disposition for reflective discussion' (QCA/DfEE 1999b: 28). Yet, at the same time, the government is encouraging the involvement in schools – and so, arguably, implicitly legitimating the activities – of private companies that have been associated with human rights infringements and anti-democratic practices in countries of the developing world. Again, it is difficult to see how teachers will be able to educate children about active citizenship, democracy and social justice without challenging the involvement in schools of commercial organisations whose own practices appear to be unjust and anti-democratic.

Finally, children are learning in an environment that is giving them little, if any, experience of democracy in action. As we have seen, schools are becoming increasingly authoritarian environments in which teachers are forced to comply with externally imposed targets, inspections and expectations. Within this environment there is little room for teachers to engage in much 'reflective discussion' *with each other* let alone encourage their children to engage in it. Schools are therefore far from operating as models of democratic practice.[34] And it is perhaps significant that in the revised national curriculum for England a distinction is drawn between the values that education 'is a route to' and the values that education 'should reflect'. It is notable that neither 'equality of opportunity for all' nor 'a healthy democracy' are listed as values that education 'should reflect'. They are merely values that education is 'a route to'. Yet, I would argue, that education cannot be a route to a healthy democracy or equality of opportunity for all, if the processes, practices and language of schooling themselves are not imbued with these values. As Deborah Meier and Paul Schwarz of Central Park East Secondary School in New York have argued:

> If the primary public responsibility and justification for tax-supported schooling is raising a generation of fellow citizens, then the school – of necessity – must be a place where students learn the habits of mind, work and heart that lie at the core of such a democracy:

34 New Labour's hostility to democratic approaches to the running of schools and to the rights of parents and children to support principles and pedagogies, which diverge from the government's preferred approach, was epitomised by the Summerhill case. Summerhill is a progressive private school run on the principles of participatory democracy and child-centred education, which gives priority to children's emotional and social development. Children are not compelled to attend lessons, do not follow the 'key stages' of the national curriculum and do not take SATs. In 1999, after repeatedly failing to respond to Ofsted's concerns that the school was providing an inadequate standard of education, the government served a notice of complaint, requiring the school to make specified improvements within a year. The school successfully appealed against this notice in a court tribunal in February 2000.

Since you cannot learn to be good at something you have never experienced – even vicariously – then it stands to reason that schools are a good place to experience what such democratic habits might be.

(Meier and Schwarz 1999: 33)

So to recap the argument of this chapter so far, New Labour has expressed a wide range of commitments in relation to education, which might be taken to suggest that the narrow economism of the Conservatives may be a thing of the past. The Blair government says it is committed to promoting social justice, a respect for cultural diversity, active citizenship, creativity, critical thinking and more open government, as well as to building a dynamic modern economy. The problem is that it is very difficult to promote these values within the context of a system of provision that subjugates teachers and children, giving them neither autonomy nor scope for creativity and that treats children as commodities, segregating them into hierarchically-tiered groupings.[35] In our compliance-oriented marketised education system there is a tendency to treat children, parents and teachers as problems to be managed and reformed rather than as active participants in making decisions about the context and content of schooling. Given these consequences, it is also difficult to imagine how third way policies are going to help resolve the problems of the state produced by Conservative post-welfarism, and it is to these problems that I now want to return.

A new educational settlement?

Can New Labour's third way be said to represent a new educational settlement? My analysis in the preceding sections of this chapter would suggest that New Labour's response to the tensions within the education system is not to dismantle the post-welfarist settlement established by the Conservatives but to refine it and attempt to

35 Although, as Michael Apple and James Beane (1999) have argued, on the basis of the experiences of schools that have succeeded in establishing democratic and critical educational practices in the context of a marketised, managerialised, under-resourced and polarised US school system, 'difficult does not mean impossible' (1999: xv). And Carrie Supple draws attention to the work of schools in the UK that the Citizenship Foundation works with, which are organised in such a way as to 'reflect the values they promote – of justice, respect, equality, rights, responsibilities and democracy, including the involvement of pupils in developing school policy' (Supple 1999: 16).

legitimate it more effectively. For, despite the rhetorical emphasis on social inclusion, widening participation and the values of 'active citizenship', we have seen that the key components of the Conservative's PWEPC are still in place and, in some cases, have been reinforced. Markets remain a key organising principle, privatisation is proceeding apace, traditionalist pedagogies are being promoted and new strategies are in place to make parents more responsible and to further managerialise, standardise, routinise and monitor the work of schools and teachers.

It is difficult to see how a perpetuation of the neo-liberal and authoritarian elements of post-welfarism is going to lead to an amelioration of the instabilities within it. For, so long as market forces and selection are allowed to operate, we are likely to see a further polarisation of educational provision (Cassidy 2000). Similarly, the problems of teacher retention, recruitment and discontent are not likely to be resolved by the increased technicisation and surveillance of teachers' work and the introduction of PRP. Indeed, a large-scale survey of primary and secondary teachers conducted three years into New Labour's first administration concluded that half of England's teachers expected to leave the profession within ten years 'mainly because they cannot stand the heavy workload, stress and bureaucracy that now accompanies a job in the classroom' (Carvel 2000; see also STRB 2000c and 2000d). And in the same year the damaging consequences for teachers' mental health of Ofsted's approach to inspection was highlighted by the well-publicised suicides of four teachers, which inquests had linked to Ofsted inspections (Mansell 2000). If polarisation and teacher discontent continue to escalate then it seems likely that New Labour policies will further exacerbate, rather than resolve, perceived problems of legitimacy and social control.

It is also questionable how far New Labour's policies will help resolve perceived problems of capital accumulation. In Chapter 6, I argued that a stressed and depleted teaching workforce is increasingly likely to be viewed as ill-equipped to produce the kinds of highly skilled future workers that are believed to be necessary for Britain to transform itself into a 'high-skill economy'. I also cited research which suggested that a high-skill economy depends upon the existence of an inclusive system of education provision (Ashton and Green 1996; see also Brown and Lauder 1996). But to create such a system would involve a more fundamental redistribution of resources than it would seem New Labour are proposing. Moreover, the forms of cognition fostered by the traditional pedagogic practices that are being promoted by New Labour, with even more vigour than their Conservative predecessors, do not correspond to the cognitive skills now being demanded by the new multinational 'knowledge-based' industries. Indeed, these traditionalist practices sit somewhat uneasily beside New Labour's *own* proposals for hastening the information and communications 'revolution' within UK schools (DfEE 1997c). According to research by Kim Seltzer and Tom Bentley (1999) what the economy needs are workers with creative problem-solving skills. Yet the fostering of creativity in schools is incompatible with a prescriptive curriculum and the 'rigid disciplinary and assessment structures that are currently in place' (Bentley and Seltzer 1999: 19). It is worthwhile reiterating here a point I made in Chapter 6: I am not suggesting that those who posit a link between creativity in education and the 'high-skill economy' are necessarily correct in their diagnosis (see Buckingham 2000). The point is that New Labour's education system is unlikely to deliver the creative skills and attitudes that a growing body of researchers (e.g., Ball 1999b; Leadbetter 1999; Seltzer and Bentley 1999) and government advisers (NACCCE 1999; Robinson 2000) as well as some of the government's own members (e.g., Smith 1998) believe are necessary for a successful 'modern' economy.

Beyond post-welfarism?

I have argued in this book that the tensions, stresses and strains within the post-welfarist settlement – first associated with Conservative education policies – are likely to inhibit the fulfilment of the diverse and conflicting expectations that informed its establishment (see Chapter 6). I have also argued that post-welfarist schooling is characterised by the production and reproduction of a number of forms of oppression and injustice (see Chapter 7). In this chapter, I have suggested that New Labour education policies are more likely to exacerbate rather than resolve the injustices, instabilities and contradictions of post-welfarism.

If my arguments have merit, we might anticipate a future scenario in which the post-welfarist education settlement is destabilised by the tensions within it and by growing levels of scepticism about its ability to deliver what is deemed to be necessary to secure economic productivity, social order and popular support for the state education system. In other words, the state will have to construct what Hay (1996) refers to as 'new modes of intervention' into the educational sphere. The new education settlement that emerges could potentially take a range of forms. As Hay has argued, new state projects are:

The subject of ideological and political contestation as competing parties vie for state power (as distinct from merely governmental power) by offering alternative visions of the future trajectory of the state to the electorate.

(Hay 1996: 98)

The contestation around the emergence of a new educational settlement may well open up a space or spaces within which it will be possible for educators, parents, and students, concerned about the injustices promoted by post-welfarist policies, to conduct struggles for social justice in education. It is beyond the scope of this book to explore what form these struggles should take, or precisely which conception of social justice they should be predicated upon. However, in thinking about what form such a politics might take, whilst we need to be alert to the danger of looking at schools in a political and economic vacuum, we need not, as Michael Apple (1996b) tells us:

embrace a fatalism that holds that it is impossible to change schools unless the social and economic relations of the wider society are transformed first. After all, such a model of analysis forgets that schools are not separate from the wider society but are part of it and participate fully in its logics and sociocultural dynamics. Struggling in schools is struggling in society . . . It is possible to create an education that highlights and opposes in practice social inequalities of many kinds, helps students to investigate how their world and their lives have come to be what they are, and seriously considers what might be done to bring about substantial alterations of this.

(Apple 1996b: 107–8)

An education of the kind that Apple envisages is dependent on the creation of non-selective, non-segregated, democratic schools, characterised by modes of association, which give students, teachers and parents the opportunity to actively participate in decision making and which enable the values of equality, creativity, critical thinking and respect for diverse cultural identities to flourish. To use the distinction drawn by Danny Burns and his colleagues in their 1994 study of local democracy, teachers, parents and students need to become 'producers' rather than 'consumers' of politics. Consumers of politics can only choose between a limited range of options presented to them or they can reject those options. They are 'rarely in a position to create' (Burns *et al.* 1994: 267). Producers of politics, on the other hand, contribute to the creation of the agenda. They decide what the choices are.

The tightness of post-welfarist forms of regulation make the kinds of struggles that Apple envisages extremely difficult in the short term. Whilst there are still teachers who are continuing to work within their classrooms to create and sustain an education that exposes and opposes social injustice, they are operating within very tightly circum-scribed boundaries. However, it may well be that if, and when, the instabilities and contradictions of post-welfarism become more pro-nounced, spaces will open up within and beyond schools in which more extensive struggles can take place to develop more socially just, non-oppressive and potentially transformative educational practices. The form that these struggles and practices ought to take now needs to be the object of serious reflection and debate.

Bibliography

ALTARF (All London Teachers Against Racism and Fascism) (1979) *Racism in Schools*, London: ALTARF.

Andrews, G. (1999) 'New Left and New Labour: modernization or a new modernity?', *Soundings* 13: 14–24.

Angus, L. (1993) 'The sociology of school effectiveness', *British Journal of Sociology of Education* 14(3): 333–45.

—— (1994) 'Sociological analysis and educational management: the social context of the self-managing school', *British Journal of Sociology of Education* 15(1): 79–92.

Apple, M. (1996a) 'Power, meaning and identity: critical sociology of education in the US', *British Journal of Sociology of Education* 17(2): 125–44.

—— (1996b) *Cultural Politics and Education*, Buckingham: Open University Press.

—— (1997) 'What postmodernists forget: cultural capital and official knowledge', in A. H. Halsey, H. Lauder, P. Brown and A. S. Wells (eds), *Education: Culture, Economy and Society*, Oxford: Oxford University Press.

Apple, M. and Beane, J. A. (eds) (1999) *Democratic Schools: Lessons from the Chalk Face*, Buckingham: Open University Press.

Arnot, M. and Weiner, G. (eds) (1987) *Gender and the Politics of Schooling*, London: Hutchinson.

Ashton, D. and Green, F. (1996) *Education, Training and the Global Economy*, Cheltenham: Edward Elgar.

Ashworth, J., Papps, I. and Thomas, B. (1988) *Increased Parental Choice: An Economic Analysis of Some Alternative Methods of Management and Finance of Education*, Warlingham: IEA Education Unit.

Bailey, P. (1999) 'Mathematics', in D. Hill and M. Cole (eds), *Promoting Equality in Secondary Schools*, London: Cassell.

Ball, S. J. (1981) *Beachside Comprehensive: A Case Study of Secondary Schooling*, Cambridge: Cambridge University Press.

—— (1987) *The Micro-Politics of the School: Towards a Theory of School Organization*, London and New York: Methuen.

—— (1990a) *Politics and Policymaking in Education: Explorations in Policy Sociology*, London: Routledge.

—— (1990b) 'Management as moral technology: a Luddite analysis', in S. J. Ball (ed.), *Foucault and Education: Disciplines and Knowledge*, London: Routledge.

—— (1997) 'Good school/bad school: paradox and fabrication', *British Journal of Sociology of Education* 18(3): 317–36.

—— (1998) 'Performativity and fragmentation in "postmodern schooling"', in J. Carter (ed.), *Postmodernity and the Fragmentation of Welfare: A Contemporary Social Policy*, London: Routledge.

—— (1999a) 'Performativities and fabrications in the education economy: towards the performative society?' Keynote address to the Australian Association of Research in Education Annual Conference, Melbourne.

—— (1999b) 'Labour, learning and the economy: a "policy sociology" perspective', *Cambridge Journal of Education* 29(2): 195–206.

Ball, S. J. and Gewirtz, S. (1997) 'Girls in the education market: choice, competition and complexity', *Gender and Education* 9(2): 207–22.

Ball, S. J., Bowe, R. and Gewirtz, S. (1994) 'Competitive schooling: values, ethics and cultural engineering', *Journal of Curriculum and Supervision* 9(4): 350–67.

—— (1995) 'Circuits of schooling: a sociological exploration of parental choice of school in social class contexts', *Sociological Review* 43(1): 52–78.

Barber, M. (1996) *The Learning Game: Arguments for an Education Revolution*, London: Victor Gollancz.

Barnard, N. and Henry, J. (2000) 'Union goes to law over new pay duty', *Times Educational Supplement*, 24 March.

Bentley, T. and Seltzer, K. (1999) 'Make room for creativity', *Times Educational Supplement*, 8 October.

Best, S. and Kellner, D. (1991) *Postmodern Theory: Critical Interrogations*, Basingstoke: Macmillan.

Blair, T. (1998) *The Third Way: New Politics for the New Century*, London: The Fabian Society.

Blunkett, D. (1999) 'Do we want to bus the middle-class?', *The Guardian*, 16 September: 21.

Boaler, J. (1994) 'When do girls prefer football to fashion? An analysis of female underachievement in relation to "realistic" mathematics contexts', *British Educational Research Journal* 20(5).

—— (1997a) 'Setting, social class and survival of the quickest', *British Educational Research Journal* 23(5): 575–95.

—— (1997b) 'When even the winners are losers: evaluating the experience of 'top set' students', *Journal of Curriculum Studies* 29(2): 165–82.

Bottery, M. (1992) *The Ethics of Educational Management*, London: Cassell.

Bourne, J., Bridges, L. and Searle, C. (1994) *Outcast England: How Schools Exclude Black Children*, London: Institute of Race Relations.

Bowe, R. and Ball, S. J., with Gold, A. (1992) *Reforming Education and Changing Schools: Case Studies in Policy Sociology*, London: Routledge.

Bowles, S. and Gintis, H. (1976) *Schooling in Capitalist America*, London: Routledge and Kegan Paul.

—— (1986) *Democracy and Capitalism*, New York: Basic Books.

Boyson, R. (1975) 'The developing case for the educational voucher', in C. B. Cox and R. Boyson (eds), *The Fight for Education*, London: Dent.

Brown, P. and Lauder, H. (1996) 'Education, globalization, and economic development', *Journal of Education Policy* 11: 1–24.

Buckingham, D. (2000) 'Creative futures? Young people, the arts and social inclusion', *Education and Social Justice* 2(3): 6–11.

Bunting, C. (1999) 'Jaded heads will be paid off', *Times Educational Supplement*, 12 November: 1.

Bunting, M. (2000) 'An eternal struggle', *The Guardian*, 3 April: 19.

Burns, D., Hambleton, R. and Hoggett, P. (1994) *The Politics of Decentralisation*, Basingstoke and London: Macmillan.

Cabinet Office (1999) *Modernising Government*, Cm 4310, London: The Stationery Office.

Caldwell, B. and Spinks, J. (1988) *The Self-Managing School*, Lewes: Falmer Press.

—— (1992) *Leading the Self-Managing School*, Lewes: Falmer Press.

Campbell, B. (1995) 'Old fogeys and angry young men: a critique of communitarianism', *Soundings*, 1: 47–64.

Campbell, R. J. and St J. Neill, S.R. (1994a) *Secondary Teachers at Work*, London: Routledge.

—— (1994b) *Curriculum Reform at Key Stage 1 – Teacher Commitment and Policy Failure*, Harlow: Longman.

Carvel, J. (2000) 'Teaching crisis – half plan to quit', *The Guardian*, 29 February: 1.

Carvel, J. and Brindle, D. (1999) 'No hiding place from change, PM warns', *The Guardian*, 21 October.

Cassidy, S. (2000) 'Market proves a diverse force', *Times Educational Supplement*, 17 March.

CBI (Confederation of British Industry) (1989) *Towards a Skills Revolution*, London: CBI.

CCCS (Centre for Contemporary Cultural Studies) (1981) *Unpopular Education*, London: Hutchinson University Library.

Chubb, J. and Moe, T. (1990) *Politics, Markets and America's Schools*, Washington, DC: The Brookings Institution.

Clarke, J. and Newman, J. (1992a) 'Managing to survive: dilemmas of changing organisational forms in the public sector', paper presented at Social Policy Association Conference, University of Nottingham, July.

—— (1992b) 'The right to manage: a second managerial revolution?', paper presented at Social Policy Association Conference, University of Nottingham, July.

―― (1997) *The Managerial State*, London: SAGE.
―― (1998) 'A modern British people? New Labour and welfare reform', paper presented at Discourse Analysis and Social Research Conference, Denmark, September.
Clarke, J., Cochrane, A. and McLaughlin, E. (1994) 'Mission accomplished or unfinished business? The impact of managerialization', in J. Clarke, A. Cochrane and E. McLaughlin (eds), *Managing Social Policy*, London: SAGE.
Clarke, J., Gewirtz, S. and McLaughlin, E. (eds) (2000) *New Managerialism, New Welfare?* London: SAGE.
Clarke, K. (1991) 'Education in a classless society', Westminster Lecture, Tory Reform Group, 12 June.
Coard, B. (1971) *How the West Indian Child is Made Educationally Sub-Normal in the British School System*, London: New Beacon Books.
Cohen, N. (1999) 'Labour's biggest fraud?' *The Observer*, 11 July: 31.
Considine, M. (1988) 'The corporate management framework as administrative science; a critique' *Australian Journal of Public Administration* 37(1): 4–18.
Cox, C. B. and Boyson, R. (eds) (1975) *The Fight for Education: Black Paper 1975*, London: Dent.
―― (eds) (1977) *Black Paper 1977*, London: Dent.
Cox, R. (1980) 'Social forces, states and world orders', *Millennium: Journal of International Studies* 10(2): 126–55.
CRE (Commission for Racial Equality) (1993) *Draft Circular on Admission Arrangements – Comments by CRE*, February, London: CRE.
Crump, S. J. (1997) 'Post-compulsory education and policy research', paper presented at research seminar, King's College London, 6 March.
Dale, R. (1989) *The State and Education Policy*, Buckingham: Open University Press.
Daunt, P. (1975) *Comprehensive Values*, London: Heinemann.
David, M. E., West, A. and Ribbens, J. (1994) *Mother's Intuition? Choosing Secondary Schools*, London: Falmer Press.
Davies, N. (1999a) 'Schools in crisis, Part 1', *The Guardian*, 14 September: 1, 4–5.
―― (1999b) 'Bias that killed the dream of equality', *The Guardian*, 15 September: 1, 4–5.
―― (1999c) 'Political coup bred educational disaster', *The Guardian*, 16 September: 1, 4–5.
―― (2000) 'Blunkett's magic tricks and the £19bn boost for education that doesn't exist', *The Guardian*, 7 March: 10–11.
Deem, R. (1980) *Schooling for Women's Work*, London: Routledge.
Deem, R., Brehony, K. and Heath, S. (1995) *Active Citizenship and the Governing of Schools*, Buckingham: Open University Press.
Denny, C. and Elliott, L. (2001) 'Labour fails to match Tory era spending', *The Guardian*, 21 March.
DES (1978) *Special Education Needs (Warnock Report)*, London: HMSO.

—— (1991) *The Parent's Charter: You and Your Child's Education*, London: HMSO.

DFE (Department for Education) (1994a) *Our Children's Education: The Updated Parent's Charter*, London: HMSO.

—— (1994b) *Pupils with Problems*, London: HMSO.

DfEE (Department for Education and Employment) (1997a) *The Road to Success*, London: Institute of Education/DfEE.

—— (1997b) *Labour Market and Skill Trends 1997/8*, London: DfEE.

—— (1997c) *Excellence in Schools*, London: The Stationery Office.

—— (1998) *Teachers: Meeting the Challenge of Change*, London: DfEE.

Douglas, M. (1987) *How Institutions Think*, London: Routledge and Kegan Paul.

du Gay, P. (1996) *Consumption and Identity at Work*, London: SAGE.

Eastwood, M. (1999) 'Some are more equal than others', *New Statesman*, 8 November.

Elliot, J. (1996) 'School effectiveness research and its critics: alternative visions of schooling', *Cambridge Journal of Education* 26(2): 199–224.

Esland, G. (1996) 'Education, training and nation-state capitalism: Britain's failing strategy', in J. Avis, M. Bloomer, G. Esland, D. Gleeson and P. Hodkinson (eds), *Knowledge and Nationhood: Education, Politics and Work*, London: Cassell.

Evans, J. and Vincent, C. (1997) 'Parental choice and special education', in R. Glatter, P. Woods and C. Bagley (eds), *Choice and Diversity in Schooling: Perspectives and Prospects*, London: Routledge.

Fergusson, R. (1994) 'Managerialism in education', in J. Clarke, A. Cochrane and E. McLaughlin (eds), *Managing Social Policy*, London: SAGE.

—— (1998) 'Choice, selection and the social construction of difference', in G. Hughes and G. Lewis (eds), *Unsettling Welfare: The Reconstruction of Social Policy*, London: Routledge.

Finegold, D. and Soskice, S. (1988) 'The failure of training in Britain: analysis and prescription', *Oxford Review of Economic Policy* 4(3).

Fitz, J., Halpin, D. and Power, S. (1993) *Education in the Market Place*, London: Kogan Page.

Foucault, M. (1988) *Politics, Philosophy, Culture: Interviews and Other Writings, 1977–1984*, New York: Routledge.

—— (1990) *The History of Sexuality: Volume 1: An Introduction*, Harmondsworth: Penguin.

Fraser, N. (1997) *Justice Interruptus: Critical Reflections on the 'Postsocialist' Condition*, New York and London: Routledge.

Friedman, M. (1955) 'The role of government in education', in R. A. Solo (ed.), *Economics and the Public Interest*, New Brunswick, New Jersey: Rutgers University Press.

—— (1962) *Capitalism and Freedom*, Chicago: Chicago University Press.

Gaster, L. (1999) 'Quality management in local government – issues and experience', unpublished paper, University of Birmingham.

Gewirtz, S. (1997) 'The education market, labour relations in schools and teacher unionism in the UK', in R. Glatter, P. A. Woods and C. Bagley (eds), *Choice and Diversity in Schooling: Perspectives and Prospects*, London: Routledge.

—— (1998) 'Conceptualizing social justice in education: mapping the territory', *Journal of Education Policy*, 13(4): 469–84.

Gewirtz, S., Ball, S. J. and Bowe, R. (1995) *Markets, Choice and Equity in Education*, Buckingham: Open University Press.

Giddens, A. (1981) *A Contemporary Critique of Historical Materialism*, Berkeley: University of California Press.

Gillborn, D. (1990) *Race, Ethnicity and Education: Teaching and Learning in Multi-ethnic Schools*, London: Unwin Hyman.

—— (1997) 'Young, black and failed by school: the market, education reform and black students', *International Journal of Inclusive Education* 1(1): 65–87.

Gillborn, D. and Gipps, C. (1996) *Recent Research on the Achievements of Ethnic Minority Pupils*, London: HMSO.

Gillborn, D. and Youdell, D. (1999) *Rationing Education: Policy, Practice, Reform and Equity*, Buckingham: Open University Press.

Glatter, R., Woods, P. and Bagley, C. (1997) 'Diversity, differentiation and hierarchy: school choice and parental preferences', in R. Glatter, P. Woods and C. Bagley (eds), *Choice and Diversity in Schooling: Perspectives and Prospects*, London: Routledge.

Grace, G. (1993) 'On the study of school leadership: beyond education management', *British Journal of Educational Studies* 41(4): 353–65.

—— (1995) *School Leadership. Beyond Education Management: An Essay in Policy Scholarship*, London and Washington: Falmer Press.

—— (1997) 'Urban education and the culture of contentment', paper presented at the Twenty-year Celebration of the MA in Urban Education, King's College London, November 1996.

Gramsci, A. (1971) *Selections from the Prison Notebooks*, London: Lawrence and Wishart.

Gray, J. (1992) 'The moral foundations of market institutions', *Choice in Welfare No. 10*, London: The Institute of Economic Affairs, Health and Welfare Unit.

Green, A. (1997) *Education, Globalization and the Nation State*, London: Macmillan.

Hall, S. (1998) 'The great moving nowhere show?, *Marxism Today*, Special Issue, November/December.

Hallam, S. and Toutounji, L. (1996) *What Do We Know about the Grouping of Pupils by Ability? A Research Review*, London: University of London, Institute of Education.

Halpin, D. (1999) 'Democracy, inclusive schooling and the politics of education', *International Journal of Inclusive Education* 3(3): 225–38.

Halpin, D. and Fitz, J. (1990) 'Researching grant-maintained schools', *Journal of Education Policy* 5(2): 167–80.

Hargreaves, A. (1994) *Changing Teachers, Changing Times: Teachers' Work and Culture in the Postmodern Age*, London: Cassell.

Hargreaves, D. (1967) *Social Relations in a Secondary School*, London: Routledge and Kegan Paul.

Harris, R. (1969) 'The larger lessons of Enfield', in C. B. Cox and A. Dyson (eds), *Black Paper Two: The Crisis in Education*, London: Critical Quarterly Society.

Harris, R. and Seldon, A. (1979) *Over-ruled on Welfare*, London: Institute of Economic Affairs.

Hatcher, R. (1998) 'Labour, Official School Improvement and Equality', *Journal of Education Policy* 13(3).

Hay, D. (1996) *Re-Stating Social and Political Change*, Buckingham: Open University Press.

Hayek, F. (1944) *The Road to Serfdom*, Chicago: University of Chicago Press.

Hayek, K. (1980) *Individualism and Economic Order*, Chicago: University of Chicago Press.

Heelas, P. and Morris, P. (eds) (1992) *The Values of the Enterprise Culture: The Moral Debate*, London: Routledge.

Henry, J. (2000) 'Pay bids increase test use', *Times Educational Supplement*, 12 May: 1.

Hill, D. and Cole, M. (eds) (1999) *Promoting Equality in Secondary Schools*, London: Cassell.

Hillgate Group (1986) *Whose Schools? A Radical Manifesto*, London: Claridge Press.

Hills, J. (1995) *Joseph Rowntree Foundation Inquiry into Income and Wealth, Volume 2*, York: Joseph Rowntree Foundation.

Hirst, J. (2000) 'Can we have some jobs, please?' *New Statesman*, 10 April.

Hood, C., Scott, C., James, O., Jones, G. and Travers, T. (1999) *Regulation inside Government: Waste-Watchers, Quality Police and Sleeze-busters*, Oxford: Oxford University Press.

Hughes, D. and Lauder, H. (1999) *Trading in Futures: Why Markets in Education Don't Work*, Buckingham: Open University Press.

Hughes, G. and Mooney, G. (1998) 'Community', in G. Hughes (ed.), *Imagining Welfare Futures*, London: Routledge.

Hunt, A. (1977) *Class and Class Structure*, London: Lawrence and Wishart.

ILO (International Labour Office) (1991) *Teachers: Challenges of the 1990s: Second Joint Meeting on Conditions of Work of Teachers*, Geneva: ILO.

Jackson, B. (1964) *Streaming: an Education System in Miniature*, London: Routledge and Kegan Paul.

Jones, K. (1999) 'English', in D. Hill and M. Cole (eds), *Promoting Equality in Secondary Schools*, London: Cassell.

Keat, R. and Abercrombie, N. (eds) (1991) *Enterprise Culture*, London: Routledge.

Kennedy, H. (1997a) *Learning Works: Widening Participation in Further Education*, Coventry: Further Education Funding Council.

—— (1997b) 'The report', *Times Educational Supplement*, 1 July.

Kirkpatrick, I. and Martinez-Lucio, M. (eds) (1995) *The Politics of Quality in the Public Sector*, London: Routledge.

Labour Party (1995) *Excellence for Everyone: Labour's Crusade to Raise Standards*, London: Labour Party.

Lacey, C. (1970) *Hightown Grammar: the School as a Social System*, Manchester: Manchester University Press.

Langan, M. (ed.) (1998) *Welfare: Needs, Rights and Risks*, London: Routledge.

Lawn, M. (1996) 'Restructuring teaching in the USA and England: moving towards the differentiated, flexible worker', *Journal of Education Policy* 10(4): 347–60.

Lawn, M. and Ozga, J. (1988) 'The educational worker? A reassessment of teachers', in J. Ozga (ed.), *Schoolwork: Approaches to the Labour Process of Teaching*, Milton Keynes: Open University Press.

Leadbetter, C. (1999) *Living on Thin Air: The New Economy*, London: Penguin.

Lee, T (1992a) 'Local management of schools and special education', in T. Booth, W. Swann, M. Masterson and P. Potts (eds), *Policies for Diversity in Education*, London: Routledge.

—— (1992b) 'Finding simple answers to complex questions: funding special needs under LMS', in G. Wallace (ed.), *Local Management of Schools: Research and Experience*, Clevedon: Multilingual Matters.

Levacic, R. (1995) *Local Management of Schools: Analysis and Practice*, Buckingham: Open University Press.

Ling, T. (2000) 'Unpacking partnership: the case of healthcare', in J. Clarke, S. Gewirtz and E. McLaughlin (eds), *New Managerialism, New Welfare?* London: SAGE.

Lowe, B. (1991) *Activity Sampling*, Hull: Humberside County Council.

Mac an Ghaill, M. (1988) *Young, Gifted and Black: Student–Teacher Relations in the Schooling of Black Youth*, Milton Keynes: Open University Press.

MacGilchrist, B. (1997) 'Reading and achievement', *Research Papers in Education* 12(2): 157–176.

McHugh, M. and McCullan, L. (1995) 'Headteacher or manager? implications for training and development', *School Organisation* 15: 23–34.

Macpherson, C. B. (1973) *Democratic Theory: Essays in Retrieval*, Oxford: Oxford University Press.

Macpherson, W. (1999) *The Stephen Lawrence Inquiry*, Cm 4262–1, London: The Stationery Office.

Mahony, P. and Hextall, I. (1997) 'Problems of accountability and reinvented government: a case study of the Teacher Training Agency', *Journal of Education Policy* 12(4): 267–84.

Mansell, W. (2000) 'Inquests link four deaths to inspection', *Times Educational Supplement*, 21 April: 1.

Marx, K. (1976) *Capital: A Critique of Political Economy, Volume 1*, translated by B. Fawkes, London: Pelican Books.

Maw, J., Fielding, M., Mitchell, P., White, J., Young, P., Ouston, J. and White, P. (1984) *Education Plc?*, London, Heinemann.

Meier, D. and Schwarz, P. (1999) 'Central Park East Secondary School: the hard part is making it happen', in M. W. Apple and J. A. Beane (eds), *Democratic Schools: Lessons from the Chalk Face*, Buckingham: Open University Press.

Menter, I., Muschamp, Y., Nicholls, P. and Ozga, J. with Pollard, A. (1997) *Work and Identity in the Primary School: a Post-Fordist Analysis*, Buckingham: Open University Press.

Miller, D. (1976) *Social Justice*, Oxford: Clarendon Press.

Mills, C. W. (1959) *The Sociological Imagination*, New York: Oxford University Press.

Mortimore, P. (1997) 'Can effective schools compensate for society?', in A. H. Halsey, H. Lauder, P. Brown and A. S. Wells (eds), *Education: Culture, Economy, Society*, Oxford: Oxford University Press.

Mortimore, P. and Whitty, G. (1997) *Can School Improvement Overcome the Effects of Disadvantage?* London: Institute of Education, University of London.

Mountfield, A. and Eastwood, N. (2000) *School Fundraising in England*, London: Directory of Social Change.

NACCCE (National Advisory Committee on Creative and Cultural Education) (1999) *All Our Futures: Creativity, Culture and Education*, (The Robinson Report), London: DfEE/DCMS.

NAS/UWT (National Association of Schoolmasters/Union of Women Teachers) (1990) *Teacher Workload Survey*, Birmingham: NAS/UWT.

—— (1991) *Teacher Workload Survey*, Birmingham: NAS/UWT.

NCE (National Commission on Education) (1995) *Success Against the Odds: Effective Schools in Disadvantaged Areas*, London: Routledge.

Newman, J. (1998) 'Managerialism and social welfare', in G. Hughes and G. Lewis (eds), *Unsettling Welfare: The Reconstruction of Social Policy*, London: Routledge.

Nielson, K. (1978) 'Class and justice', in J. Arthur and W. Shaw (eds), *Justice and Economic Distribution*, Englewood Cliffs, New Jersey: Prentice-Hall.

Noden, P. (2000) 'Rediscovering the impact of marketisation: dimensions of social segregation in England's secondary schools, 1994–99', *British Journal of Sociology of Education* 21(3): 371–90.

Oakes, J. (1990) *Multiplying Inequalities: the Effects of Race, Social Class and Tracking on Opportunities to Learn Mathematics and Science*, Santa Monica, California: Rand Corporation.

Ofsted (Office for Standards in Education) (2000) *Inspecting Schools: Handbook for Inspecting Secondary Schools*, London: The Stationary Office, (www.official-documents.co.uk,document/ofsted/inspect/secondary/29503.htm).

Osler, A. (1999) 'The Crick Report: difference, equality and racial justice', paper presented at ESRC Seminar on 'Human Rights, Democracy and Lifelong Learning', University of Leicester, 15 October.

Ozga, J. (1995) 'Markets, management and the manufacture of consent in primary schools', paper presented to Second Comparative Education Policy Seminar: Sweden and the UK, School of Education, King's College London, April.

—— (2000) 'New Labour, new teachers', in J. Clarke, S. Gewirtz and E. McLaughlin (eds), *New Managerialism/New Welfare?* London: SAGE.

—— (ed.) (1988) *Schoolwork: Approaches to the Labour Process of Teaching*, Milton Keynes: Open University Press.

Penney, D. and Evans, J. (1992) 'From "policy" to "practice": the development and implementation of the National Curriculum for physical education', paper presented at CEDAR International Conference, University of Warwick, 10–12 April.

Piachaud, D. (1999) 'Progress on poverty: will Blair deliver on eliminating child poverty?', *New Economy* 6(3), September: 154–60.

Plant , R. (1992) 'Enterprise in its place: the moral limits of markets', in P. Heelas and P. Morris (eds), *The Values of the Enterprise Culture: The Moral Debate*, London: Routledge.

Plewis, I. (1998) 'Inequalities, targets and Education Action Zones', *New Economy* 5.

Pollard, A., Broadfoot, P., Croll, P., Osborn, M. and Abbott, D. (1994) *Changing English Primary Schools? The Impact of the Education Reform Act at Key Stage One*, London: Cassell.

Poulantzas, N. (1973) *Political Power and Social Classes*, London: New Left Books.

—— (1978) *State, Power, Socialism*, London: New Left Books.

Power, M. (1997) *The Audit Society: Rituals of Verification*, Oxford: Oxford University Press.

QCA/DfEE (Qualifications and Curriculum Authority/Department for Education and Employment) (1999a) *The Revised National Curriculum*, London: QCA.

—— (1999b) *The Review of the National Curriculum in England: The Secretary of State's Proposals*, London: QCA.

Raab, C. (1991) 'Education policy and management: contemporary changes in Britain', paper presented to International Institute of Administrative Sciences, Copenhagen, July.

—— (1994) 'Where we are now: reflections on the sociology of education policy', in D. Halpin and B. Troyna (eds), *Researching Education Policy: Ethical and Methodological Issues*, London: Falmer Press.

Ranson, S. (1990) 'From 1944 to 1988: education, citizenship and democracy', in M. Flude and M. Hammer (eds), *The Education Reform Act 1988: Its Origins and Implications*, Lewes: Falmer Press.

Rawls, J. (1972) *A Theory of Justice*, Oxford: Clarendon Press.

Reay, D. (1998) 'Micro-politics in the 1990s: staff relationships in secondary schooling', *Journal of Education Policy* 13(2): 179–96.

Reynolds, D. and Packer, A. (1992) 'School effectiveness and school improvement in the 1990s', in D. Reynolds and P. Cuttance (eds), *School Effectiveness: Research, Policy and Practice*, London: Cassell.

Robertson, S. (1996) 'Teachers' work, restructuring and postfordism: constructing the new "professionalism"', in I. Goodson and A. Hargreaves (eds), *Teachers' Professional Lives*, London: Falmer Press.

Robertson, S. and Soucek, V. (1991) 'Changing social realities in Australian schools: a study of teachers' perceptions and experiences of current reforms', paper presented at the Comparative and International Education Society conference in Pittsburgh, Pennsylvania.

Robinson, G. (2000) *The Creativity Imperative: Investing in the Arts in the 21st Century*, London: Arts Council of England.

Robinson, P. (1997) *Literacy, Numeracy and Economic Performance*, London: Centre for Economic Performance, London School of Economics.

Roemer, J. (1982) *A General Theory of Exploitation and Class*, Cambridge, Massachusetts: Harvard University Press.

Rose, N. (1996) 'Governing "advanced" liberal democracies', in A. Barry, T. Osborne and N. Rose (eds), *Foucault and Political Reason: Liberalism, Neo-liberalism and Rationalities of Government*, London: UCL.

Salmon, J. (1997) 'Ill-health blamed for exodus of staff', *Times Educational Supplement*, 12 September.

Saraga, E. (ed.) (1998) *Embodying the Social. Constructions of Difference*, London: Routledge.

Scott, D. (1997) 'The missing hermeneutical dimension in mathematical modelling of school effectiveness', in M. Barber and J. White (eds), *Perspectives on School Effectiveness and School Improvement*, London: University of London, Institute of Education.

Seltzer, K. and Bentley, T. (1999) *The Creative Age*, London: Demos.

SEU (Social Exclusion Unit) (1998) *Truancy and Social Exclusion: Report by the Social Exclusion Unit*, Cm. 3957, London: The Stationery Office.

Sexton, S. (1987) *Our Schools: A Radical Policy*, Warlingham: Institute of Economic Affairs, Education Unit.

Slavin, R.E. (1996) *Education for All*, Lisse: Swets and Zeitlinger.

Smith, A. (1937) *The Wealth of Nations*, Modern Library Edition, New York: Random House.

Smith, C. (1998) *Creative Britain*, London: Faber & Faber.

Smyth, J. and Shacklock, G. (1998) *Re-Making Teaching: Ideology, Policy and Practice*, London: Routledge.

Stewart, J. and Ranson, S. (1988) 'Management in the public domain', *Public Money and Management*, spring/summer: 13–19.

Stoll, L. (1995) 'The complexity and challenge of ineffective schools', paper presented to the European Conference on Educational Research and the Annual Conference of the British Educational Research Association, Bath.

Stoll, L. and Fink, D. (1996) *Changing Our Schools: Linking School Effectiveness and School Improvement*, Buckingham: Open University Press.

Storey, J. (1992) *Developments in the Management of Human Resources*, Oxford: Blackwell.

STRB (School Teachers' Review Body) (1996) *Managing Teachers' Workloads*, London: Office of Manpower Economics.

—— (2000a) *Teachers' Workloads Diary Survey*, London: Office of Manpower Economics.

—— (2000b) *A Study of Teachers' Workloads*, London: Office of Manpower Economics.

—— (2000c) *Recruitment and Retention of Classroom Teachers*, Manchester: Whitmuir.

—— (2000d) *The Recruitment and Retention of Classroom Teachers*, London: IRS Research.

Sukhnandan, L. and Lee, B. (1998) *Streaming, Setting and Grouping by Ability*, Slough: NFER.

Supple, C. (1999) 'The Citizenship Foundation – our ideals for citizenship education', *Multicultural Teaching* 18(1) Autumn: 16–19.

Thomas, J. (1993) *Doing Critical Ethnography*, Newbury Park, California: SAGE.

Thomas, S. and Mortimore, P. (1996) 'Comparison of value added models for secondary school effectiveness', *Research Papers in Education* 11(1): 5–33.

Thornton, K. (2000) 'Budget cash can cut class sizes, heads told', *Times Educational Supplement*, 14 April.

Thrupp, M. (1998) 'The art of the possible: organising and managing high and low socio-economic schools', *Journal of Education Policy* 13(2): 197–219.

—— (1999) *Schools Making a Difference: Let's be Realistic! School Mix, School Effectiveness and the Social Limits of Reform*, Buckingham: Open University Press.

Tomlinson, S. (1987) 'Curriculum option choices in multi-ethnic schools', in B. Troyna (ed.), *Racial Inequality in Education*, London: Tavistock.

Troyna, B., Hatcher, R. and Gewirtz, D. (1993) *Local Management of Schools and Racial Equality*, London: Commission for Racial Equality.

Waine, B. (2000) 'Paying for performance', in J. Clarke, S. Gewirtz and E. McLaughlin (eds), *New Managerialism, New Welfare?*, London: SAGE.

Watkins, P. (1992) *Class, the Labour Process and Work: Focus on Education*, Geelong: Deakin University Press.

White, J. (1997) 'Philosophical perspectives on school effectiveness and improvement', in M. Barber and J. White (eds), *Perspectives on School Effectiveness and School Improvement*, London: Institute of Education, University of London.

Whitty, G. (1997) 'Social theory and education policy: the legacy of Karl Mannheim', *British Journal of Sociology of Education* 18(2): 149–63.

—— (1998) 'New Labour, education and disadvantage', *Education and Social Justice* 1(1): 2–8.

Whitty, G., Edwards, T. and Gewirtz, S. (1993) *Specialisation and Choice in Urban Education: the City Technology College Experiment*, London: Routledge.

Whitty, G., Power, S. and Halpin, D. (1998) *Devolution and Choice in Education: The School, the State and the Market*, Buckingham: Open University Press.

Williams, F. (1991) 'The welfare state as part of a racially structured and patriarchal capitalism', in M. Loney, R. Bocock, J. Clarke, A. Cochrane, P. Graham and M. Wilson (eds), *The State or the Market*, London: SAGE.

Williams, R. (1962) *The Long Revolution*, Harmondsworth: Penguin.

Willms, J. D. (1996) 'School choice and community segregation: findings from Scotland', in A. C. Kerckchoff (ed.), *Generating Social Stratification: towards a New Research Agenda*, Boulder, Colorado and Oxford: Westview Press.

Wintour, P. and Bright, M. (1997) 'Blunkett teaches "can-do" concept', *The Observer*, 6 July.

Woods, P. and Jeffrey, B. (1998) 'Choosing positions: living the contradictions of Ofsted', *British Journal of Sociology of Education* 19(4): 547–70.

Woods, P., Bagley, C. and Glatter, R. (1998) *School Choice and Competition: Markets in the Public Interest?* Buckingham: Open University Press.

Woods, P., Jeffrey, B., Troman, G. and Boyle, M. (1997) *Restructuring Schools, Reconstructing Teachers: Responding to Changes in the Primary School*, Buckingham: Open University Press.

Wright, E. O. (1985) *Classes*, London: Verso.

—— (1988) 'Exploitation, identity and class structure: a reply to my critics', *Critical Sociology* 15(1): 91–110.

Yeatman, A. (1993) 'Corporate managerialism and the shift from the welfare to the competition state', *Discourse* 13(2): 10–17.

Young, I. M. (1990) *Justice and the Politics of Difference*, Princeton, New Jersey: Princeton University Press.

Young, M. F. D. (1971) *Knowledge and Control: New Directions for the Sociology of Education*, London: Collier-Macmillan.

Zeitlin, M. (ed.) (1980) *Classes, Class Conflict and the State*, Cambridge: Winthrop.

Appendix

Notes on the research methods deployed in the two empirical studies informing Part I

Chapter 3 draws on data collected from 'Northwark Park' school, one of fourteen schools that participated in the ESRC-funded Markets in Secondary Education Project (the 'Markets Study'). The study was designed to explore the operation and effects of parental choice and market forces in education, focusing on three competitive clusters of schools in three geographically contiguous LEAs in London. For full details of the research methods used in this project see Gewirtz *et al.* (1995: 13–18). The Northwark Park data-set, upon which Chapter 3 draws, consists of 16 in-depth interviews with staff and governors at the school, observations of recruitment evenings and days for parents, in-service training days for teachers, governors' meetings and meetings of the committee established to boost student recruitment, school brochures, and planning and report documentation.

The 16 interviewees were chosen to represent a cross-section of teachers and governors, including: the special needs teacher because previous research (e.g., Bowe *et al.* 1992) had indicated that students with special needs were particularly vulnerable in the market place; the head of Year 7 who was responsible for primary liaison because we were aware that he had a potentially key role to play in student recruitment and the marketing of the school; and the two union representatives (from the NUT and NAS/UWT) because we were interested in union activity and the labour relations perspective on events within the schools that these informants could provide (see Gewirtz 1997). We also attempted to ensure that we had within our sample a range in terms of length of experience and position of responsibility. In addition to the cross-sectional sampling, we interviewed staff who, on the basis of informal conversations, their contributions to school meetings and/or recommendation from other members of staff, we believed would have particularly useful things to say, in terms of our developing analyses, and who seemed especially thoughtful, reflexive and articulate.

Chapters 2, 4, and 5 draw on data collected as part of the ESRC-funded study of Schools, Cultures and Values (the 'Values Study'). The research was based upon the production of in-depth, ethnographic case studies of four very different secondary schools. The schools were selected in order to highlight contrasting features in terms of market position, responses to the market, socio-cultural differences in the composition of student and governing bodies, differences in the history and constitution of management teams, and in the institutional 'visions' and mission statements of schools.

Across the four schools, 101 ethnographic interviews were carried out with a cross-section of staff and governors. The cross-section was determined mainly by the following criteria: length of experience, subject and position of responsibility. Administrative as well as teaching staff were included. As in the Markets Study, we also interviewed staff who appeared to have novel perspectives and staff who seemed especially thoughtful. Breakdowns of the Values Study interview sample, by role in school and length of service, are provided in Tables 4 and 5.

In addition, 94 observational visits were made to the schools. A breakdown of observations is provided in Table 6. Through observations we accessed data on management styles and practices, the nature of decision making in the schools, social relations, language use, and the values and priorities that fed into and informed planning and day-to-day decision making. Our observation included some shadowing of headteachers and deputies. This gave us a feel for the different ways these senior managers acted out their roles on a day-to-day

Table 4 Interviews in Values Study schools

Category of staff/governor	No. of interviews
Headteacher	9
Deputy heads	11
Senior teachers	7
Heads of department	26
Heads of year	10
Other teachers	29
Administrative staff	6
Governors	3*
Total	**101†**

* Plus 3 teacher governors, included in other categories.
† There were 96 interviewees – 5 were interviewed twice.

Table 5 Values Study interviewees by length of service

	pre-1972	1972–79	1980–87	1988–91	1992–95	Non-teacher	Information not elicited	Total
In teaching	13	24	20	12	12	9	6	96
In case-study school	4	8	21	33	25	–	5	96

Table 6 Values Study observations

Observations	No. of visits
Days shadowing managers	7
In-service training days	12
Senior management meetings	25
Heads of year/heads of department meetings	11
Department meetings	3
Staff meetings	10
Governors' meetings	17
Meetings for parents	9
Total	**94**

basis as they moved across and between different contexts within the schools. In addition to interviews and observation, we also collected documentation – prospectuses, minutes, policies, development plans. Taken alongside the other data sources, these helped us to build up a picture of language use, values, priorities and marketing activities.

In both studies we used aide-mémoirs to guide the interviews. As far as possible, we allowed respondents to talk about issues which they felt to be of particular significance. However, there were some matters that we tried to cover with all staff, such as recruitment issues in the Markets Study and changes in classroom practice in the Values Study. The formal interviews were complemented by a series of informal staffroom conversations. These were particularly useful for eliciting perspectives on day-to-day events in the schools as they occurred and for gathering data from a wider sample of respondents than was possible through formal interviewing.

Index